Small Steps, Great Gain: Adding Years to Your Lifespan

DAVID K. LOPEZ (Ph.D)

Introduction:

Welcome to a transformative journey of small steps and extraordinary gains. In a world inundated with grand promises and quick fixes, we often overlook the incredible power of simplicity. But what if I told you that the key to a longer, healthier life lies not in drastic measures but in the subtle art of small steps?

In 'Small Steps, Great Gains: Adding Years to Your Lifespan,' we invite you to embark on a journey of self-discovery and empowerment. This book is not just about adding years to your life, but about infusing life into your years. It's about embracing the concept that tiny changes, when consistently applied, can yield remarkable results.

Each page of this book is filled
with practical wisdom, inspiring
stories, and evidence-backed
strategies to help you make
small, sustainable changes that
will positively impact your
health and well-being. Our aim is
to guide you through the maze of
information and provide you
with simple, actionable steps that
can be seamlessly integrated into
your everyday life.
No matter where you are on your
wellness journey, whether you're
just starting out or looking to
fine-tune your existing habits,
'Small Steps, Great Gains' is your
compass. We believe that
everyone deserves to experience
the profound benefits of a
healthier lifestyle, and we're here
to show you how to achieve it,
one small step at a time.
Throughout the chapters that
follow, we'll explore various
areas of your life where small
changes can make a big
difference. From nutrition and
physical activity to sleep, stress
management, and preventive
healthcare, we'll delve into the
essential components of a well-
rounded, vibrant life. Each

chapter is designed to provide you with practical insights, actionable strategies, and the motivation to take that first step towards a healthier, more fulfilling future.

But this book is not just about the science of health; it's about the art of transformation. It's about embracing the joy of progress, celebrating small victories, and cultivating a mindset of self-compassion and resilience. We'll share inspiring stories of individuals who have embraced small steps and witnessed extraordinary gains in their own lives. Their journeys will inspire you, reminding you that change is possible and that every small action matters.

So, are you ready to rewrite your story? Are you ready to let go of the all-or-nothing mindset and embrace the power of small steps? Together, we'll navigate the challenges, debunk the myths, and lay the foundation for a healthier, more vibrant future. Turn the page, take that first small step, and let 'Small Steps, Great Gains: Adding Years to Your Lifespan' be your guide on this transformative journey. It's time to unlock the immense potential within you and create a life filled with vitality, purpose, and extraordinary gains

CHAPTER 1

WHY SMALL CHANGES?
Tiny adjustments to our medical care can have a big impact on how long we live and how well we are in general. An examination of how minor adjustments to several health factors can result in a longer lifespan is provided below:

1. **Nutrition**: Making little dietary changes can increase longevity and improve health outcomes. For instance, consuming fewer processed foods and added sugars while increasing the amount of fruits, vegetables, whole grains, and lean proteins in our diets can help us maintain a healthy weight, fend against chronic diseases like diabetes and

heart disease, and improve our general well-being.

2. **Physical Activity**: Physical activity, even in modest amounts, can have a big impact on lifespan. We may improve our cardiovascular health, strengthen our muscles and bones, manage our weight, lower our chance of developing chronic diseases, and improve our mental health by choosing the stairs over the elevator, taking short walks, or including shorter exercise sessions in our daily routine.

3. **Sleep**: Making sleep a top priority can significantly affect our health and longevity. Small changes can help to promote restorative sleep, improve cognitive function, support immune function, and lower the risk of chronic conditions like obesity, diabetes, and cardiovascular disease. These changes include creating a relaxing

bedtime routine, sticking to a regular sleep schedule, optimizing the sleep environment (e.g., reducing noise and light), and practicing good sleep hygiene.

4. **Stress management**: Making minor lifestyle adjustments to reduce stress will help you live a longer life. Blood pressure can be lowered, immune function can be improved, the risk of mental health disorders can be decreased, and general well-being can be improved by incorporating stress reduction techniques like deep breathing exercises, mindfulness meditation, spending time in nature, engaging in hobbies, and fostering social connections.

5. **Alcohol and Tobacco Use**: Making the decision to stop drinking alcohol or quitting smoking, even in tiny doses, can have a major positive impact on health outcomes and

lifetime. The risk of several malignancies, cardiovascular disorders, respiratory issues, and liver ailments can be decreased by making these modifications.

6. **Screen Time and Sedentary Behavior**: Reducing sedentary behavior and setting time limits on screen use, particularly for activities like prolonged TV watching and excessive use of electronic gadgets, can extend longevity. It is possible to enhance cognitive performance, lower the risk of obesity, and improve metabolic health by incorporating brief breaks for stretching or modest physical activity throughout the day. Passive screen time can also be substituted with mentally stimulating activities.

7. **Preventive Health**care: Regular preventive healthcare measures, such as getting regular

checkups, screenings, and vaccinations, can identify health risks at an early stage or completely prevent them. Small actions like keeping up with prescribed immunizations, making frequent checkups, and tracking health metrics (such blood pressure and cholesterol levels) can help with early disease intervention and disease prevention, which will ultimately result in a longer and better life.

It's crucial to remember that even while each minor adjustment can appear unimportant on its own, the cumulative effect of various changes over time might result in major health advantages and lengthen lifetime. We have the capacity to improve our overall health, prevent chronic diseases, and prolong the quality of our lives as we age by implementing consistent and long-lasting adjustments to our daily routines and behaviors.

We will go into comprehensive explanations of these pieces as we go deeper into them.

CHAPTER 2

CARDIOVASCULAR HEALTH

Your heart and blood vessels' general health is referred to as cardiovascular health. It involves the cardiovascular system's normal operation, which is in charge of pumping blood throughout your body.

By lowering the risk of cardiovascular diseases and other related consequences, maintaining cardiovascular health can greatly lengthen lifetime. Here are a few ways that maintaining cardiovascular health makes it possible to live longer and in better health:

- **Lower risk of heart disease**: You can lower your risk of getting heart disease by leading a healthy lifestyle that includes regular exercise, a balanced diet, and quitting smoking. As a result, there is a lower chance of having heart attacks, angina, and other potentially fatal cardiac events.

- **Lower risk of stroke**: Strokes, which happen when the blood supply to the brain is interrupted, are less likely to occur in those who have good cardiovascular health. Strokes can result in fatalities or very serious disabilities. You can reduce your risk of stroke by controlling your blood pressure, cholesterol, and living a healthy lifestyle.
- **Preventing additional cardiovascular complications**: Heart failure, peripheral artery disease, and arrhythmias (abnormal heart rhythms) are just a few of the issues that can result from cardiovascular disorders. You can lessen the risk of having these illnesses and their related hazards by

maintaining cardiovascular health.

- **Improved overall health**: Cardiovascular health and general wellbeing are closely related. You are taking care of other parts of your body as well by putting your cardiovascular health first. Regular physical activity and a nutritious diet can help maintain a healthy weight, increase bone density, strengthen the immune system, and improve mental health, all of which are factors in living a longer and healthier life.

- **The improved quality of life**: Maintaining cardiovascular health enables you to engage in regular activities and physical activity without difficulty. Your stamina, energy, and general vitality are improved. You can lead an active lifestyle, pursue your interests, and spend quality time with loved ones by avoiding cardiovascular illnesses and their complications.

When we discuss cardiovascular health, we are interested in a number of elements that support the heart and blood vessels' ideal operation. Although there are many of these factors, we will just go into detail about three of them. They consist of:

1. Blood pressure
2. Heart health.
3. Level of cholesterol.

1. **Blood pressure.**

High blood pressure, sometimes referred to as hypertension, is becoming a concern for more people. It is frequently referred to as the quiet executioner because it frequently shows no symptoms prior to actually injuring the body. Hypertension can in every way lead to coronary disease, stroke, and other dangerous clinical issues. Fortunately, there are effective ways to reduce circulatory strain and the likelihood of these problems.

You will soon discover helpful advice and methods for changing your lifestyle that can help you reduce your circulatory strain and improve your general well-being. This book is a wonderful resource that can aid you whether you're trying to manage hypertension that is already present or prevent it.

Let's get started.

How does blood pressure work?

Blood pressure, also referred to as pulse, is the force of blood pushing against the body's internal walls. A basic assessment reveals how well our organs and tissues are supplied with oxygen and other nutrients via the heart and veins. Maintaining a steady pulse is important for overall cardiovascular health and ensuring proper blood flow throughout the body.

There are a few phrases that must be covered before continuing. especially the ones who will find them intriguing to hear. As follows:

BLOOD PRESSURE, SYSTOLIC

The top figure in a blood pressure reading, or systolic blood pressure, indicates the pressure placed on the artery walls when the heart contracts and pumps blood into the circulatory system. It displays the heart's maximum force generated throughout each heartbeat.

The left ventricle of the heart contracts, forcing oxygenated blood into the arteries, feeding the body's organs and tissues with vital nutrients and oxygen. Systolic blood pressure is calculated as a result of the force that causes an increase in pressure against the artery walls.

Systolic blood pressure is significant because it shows how well the heart pumps blood and how robust the cardiovascular system is overall. It is affected by a number of variables, such as the heart's ability to contract forcefully, the amount of blood being pumped, and the flexibility and resistance of the arteries.

Systolic pressure is the greater number in a blood pressure reading, and diastolic pressure is the lower number. For instance, the systolic pressure is **120 mmHg** in a blood pressure reading of 120/80 mmHg.

Systolic blood pressure is measured by medical

practitioners to evaluate how well the heart and circulatory system are working. Uncontrolled hypertension (high blood pressure), which can cause major health issues like heart disease, stroke, and renal damage, can be identified by persistently high systolic blood pressure.

For cardiovascular health, systolic blood pressure must be kept within a reasonable range. Modifying one's lifestyle to include regular exercise, a healthy diet, managing weight, and reducing stress can help regulate and maintain ideal systolic blood pressure levels. For the purpose of identifying and managing any systolic blood pressure irregularities, regular blood pressure monitoring and consultation with a healthcare expert are essential.

BLOOD PRESSURE, DIASTOLIC

The bottom figure in a blood pressure reading, or diastolic blood pressure, indicates the pressure placed on the artery walls when the heart is at rest in between contractions. It denotes the lowest force or pressure in the arteries throughout the heart's pumping cycle's rest phase.

The heart slows down and fills up with blood during diastole to get ready for the next contraction. When the heart is at rest, the diastolic blood pressure measurement represents the pressure in the arteries.

Diastolic blood pressure is significant because it tells us how much pressure is in the arteries at rest, which tells us how much blood flow is blocked in the peripheral circulation and how easily the arteries may relax and permit continuous blood flow.

The flexibility of the arteries, the amount of blood in the arteries, and the resistance to blood flow from smaller blood vessels (arterioles) are some of the factors that affect diastolic pressure.

The lower number in a blood pressure reading is the diastolic pressure; the larger number is the systolic pressure. For instance, the diastolic pressure is 80 mmHg when the blood pressure is 120/80 mmHg.

Diastolic blood pressure is closely monitored by medical practitioners since it sheds light on the condition of the cardiovascular system. Diastolic blood pressure that is consistently higher than normal might be a sign of hypertension (high blood pressure), which can put stress on the heart and result in complications like heart disease, stroke, and kidney issues.

Stage 1 of hypertension.

In hypertension Stage 1, sometimes referred to as high blood pressure Stage 1, your arteries are continually being pushed against by more force than is normal. When your blood pressure readings fall inside a predetermined range, this issue is often diagnosed.

Your blood pressure readings for Stage 1 hypertension will normally show a systolic pressure (the top number) between 130 and 139 mmHg and a diastolic pressure (the bottom number) between 80 and 89 mmHg. These data reveal that during both the contraction and relaxation phases of your heart's pumping cycle, the pressure in your blood arteries is raised.

Even though your blood pressure is somewhat elevated if you have Stage 1 hypertension, you should still address and control it. Your cardiovascular system may be strained by uncontrolled high blood pressure, which raises your risk of heart disease, stroke, and other consequences.

Stage 2 hypertension

A significant medical disease known as hypertension stage 2, sometimes referred to as high blood pressure stage 2, is characterized by persistently high blood pressure readings. The force that the blood applies to the artery walls as it travels through them is known as blood pressure. Blood pressure values in stage 2 hypertension are higher than average and fall within a predetermined range. It is specifically described as having a systolic blood pressure (the top number) or a diastolic blood pressure (the bottom number) that is continuously higher than 140 mm Hg throughout time.

High blood pressure raises the risk of numerous health issues by putting additional load on the organs and arteries. It can eventually result in kidney issues, heart disease, a stroke, and other severe illnesses.

HIGH PRESSURE CRISIS

A serious, sometimes fatal disease known as a hypertensive crisis is characterized by an abrupt, extremely high rise in blood pressure. It is regarded as a medical emergency that needs to be attended to right away.

however there are two different kinds.

1. urgent hypertension
2. Hypertensive crisis

Extremely high blood pressure values are present in hypertensive urgency, but no immediate organ damage is seen. Systolic and diastolic blood pressure are often both above 180 and 120 mm Hg, respectively. Severe headaches, breathing difficulties, nosebleeds, and anxiety are possible symptoms. To lower the blood pressure and stop it from rising to the point of becoming a hypertensive emergency, immediate medical intervention is still required.

Emergency hypertension

This condition causes a sudden rise in blood pressure that causes immediate organ damage. The brain, heart, kidneys, and eyes are just a few of the organs that it may influence. Readings of blood pressure frequently reach 180/120 mm Hg and are abnormally high. Severe headaches, chest discomfort, shortness of breath, confusion, vision issues, seizures, and even loss of consciousness are possible symptoms.

Emergency hypertensive situations necessitate prompt medical attention, usually in a hospital environment. The main objective is to progressively lower blood pressure while avoiding organ damage. For hours or days, intravenous medicines are typically used to lower the blood pressure to a safe level. During this time, it's important to keep a close eye on organ function and vital signs.

Hypotension.

Low blood pressure, sometimes referred to as hypotension, is a medical condition marked by unnaturally low blood pressure values. The force that blood applies to the artery walls as it travels through the body is known as blood pressure. When there is hypotension, the organs and tissues do not receive enough oxygen and nourishment.

Dizziness, lightheadedness, fainting, blurred vision, weariness, and confusion are typical signs of hypotension. Dehydration, drug side effects, hormonal imbalances, heart issues, or underlying medical diseases are just a few of the causes.

Hypotension that is mild may not need treatment, but hypotension that is severe or chronic may need medical attention. Among the possible courses of action for treatment are addressing the underlying cause, upping hydration and salt consumption, raising blood pressure with medication, and wearing compression stockings to enhance blood flow.

WHEN IS THE HIGH AND LOW OF YOUR BLOOD PRESSURE?

I didn't say anything about when your blood pressure is low and high above.

Systolic pressure and diastolic pressure are the two numbers used to calculate blood pressure. Diastolic pressure is the force on the artery walls when the heart is at rest in between beats, whereas systolic pressure is the force on the artery walls when the heart contracts. Systolic pressure over diastolic pressure is the usual way to express blood pressure, for example, 120/80 mmHg.

The American Heart Association (AHA) divides blood pressure into the following groups:

Hypotension: is the medical term for low blood pressure.

Normal: below 120/80 mmHg Systolic between 120 and 129 mmHg and diastolic under 80 mmHg are considered elevated.

Stage 1 hypertension: Systolic pressure of 130-139 mmHg or diastolic pressure of 80-89 mmHg.

Stage 2 hypertension: Systolic pressure of at least 140 mmHg or diastolic pressure of at least 90 mmHg a hypertensive emergency > 180 mmHg in the systolic or over 120 mmHg in the diastolic

It's crucial to remember that these categories are only broad recommendations, and that each person's unique situation and medical history should be taken into account. Given that blood pressure can vary throughout the day due to a number of reasons, a single high reading may not always signify hypertension. Numerous readings taken at various periods are often required for the diagnosis of hypertension.

How do these two individuals manage their hypertension?

I always tell those who are struggling with high blood pressure that it's not the end of the world.

Claire D'Andrea was recently interviewed by **MU/PD** to discuss her experience with high blood pressure. Here is her tale. Her tale is told to uplift and inspire you.

MU/PD: How were you made aware of your high blood pressure?

Claire: At a moment in my life when I was under a lot of stress, I was diagnosed with high blood pressure. A few months before, my husband's company had closed, and he was consequently laid off. With our three children, we made the decision to move to San Diego. I had to balance working as a nurse, caring for my son and two daughters, and household chores like cooking, cleaning, and taking the kids to extracurricular activities because my husband had relocated to California a year before we had.

I started seeing stars in my vision that looked like kaleidoscopes when I was 42 years old and I was driving my daughter to ice skating practice. My blood pressure was 210/120 when I saw the doctor on that particular day, as opposed to a normal reading of 120/80. After receiving a diagnosis of high blood pressure, I worked with my doctor to adopt a healthy lifestyle and follow my recommended meds.

MU/PD: Has your elevated blood pressure resulted in further health issues?

Claire: I was walking our dog when I felt an excruciating pain between my shoulder blades about six months after my kids and I relocated to California to join my husband. My primary care doctor's visit ended with a normal EKG and a recommendation for a cardiologist. I underwent a stress test there that only required three minutes of treadmill walking since I needed nitro and oxygen to recuperate. I visited the hospital three days later for a coronary angiography in order to have a stent inserted to improve blood flow through my narrow or clogged arteries. At the time, my hypertension was the only risk factor for developing heart disease.

How has your health altered recently, MU/PD?

Claire: I've gained much more control over my health since being diagnosed with high blood pressure and receiving a coronary artery stent by concentrating on my risk factors. It was crucial for me to learn coping mechanisms for emotions and stress in order to get healthier. How did I manage this? I obtained my certification in therapeutic touch, share my knowledge of stress management with others, routinely practice yoga to strengthen my body and mind, practice regular meditation, and keep a blog.

By directing a WomenHeart Support Group in my neighborhood, which I have done for ten years, I also assist other women who suffer from high blood pressure, heart disease, and other cardiovascular problems. I speak publicly about heart disease for WomenHeart and distribute literature and Red Bags of Courage at health fairs to inform other women and empower them to take care of themselves.

Isn't it a fascinating tale?

Here is yet another inspiring tale. an interview with ROLANDA PERKINS conducted by the MU/PD.

MU/PD: How were you made aware of your excessive blood pressure?

Rolanda: My heart attack in 2005 was partially brought on by excessive blood pressure.

Despite having multiple risk factors, I was completely unaware that I had heart disease prior to the incident.

Nearly 70% of individuals who experience a heart attack also have excessive blood pressure. How did you find that experience?

Rolanda: It was an extremely spooky situation. I had been under a lot of stress working the third shift and organizing a surprise birthday party for my sister before I had my heart attack. I blamed the stress for a few days' worth of headaches that I thought were migraines. To see if taking painkillers for migraines would help, I did. I can see now that my body was trying to communicate with me.

We had a barbecue with friends and family the day following the surprise celebration. Afterward, as I was mopping and cleaning up, I suddenly experienced a severe discomfort in my chest. I ignored that agony, but about 3:30 in the morning it woke me up, and I was sent to the emergency department.

After describing my symptoms to the triage nurse, I didn't have to wait until I was in the emergency department. After being taken to the back for medical attention, I was informed that I was experiencing a heart attack. A narrow tube with a tiny balloon on the end was threaded through a blood vessel close to my heart and inflated to enlarge the artery and restore blood flow to my heart and body. This procedure is known as an angioplasty. High blood pressure was one of the diagnoses I received before being discharged from the hospital.

Do you have any conditions that could put you at risk for high blood pressure or a heart attack?

Rolanda: My life's stress level played a significant role. My parents, brother, and sister all have high blood pressure, and it runs in the family. My way of life was also an issue. I frequently ate more sodium than I should have because I didn't pay attention to how much was in the things I ate.

How did you alter these risk variables to better manage your blood pressure, MU/PD?
Rolanda: There are other risk variables that I have no control over, such as color, age, gender, and family history. But I was aware that I had complete control over my lifestyle, particularly my eating and exercise habits.

For instance, I used to eat a can of beefaroni with garlic bread and a salad with Italian dressing for dinner before having a heart attack. I didn't understand how much sodium was in the cuisine; just one serving of beefaroni contains about half of the recommended daily intake!

Knowing this, I started eating better food in smaller portions, walking on a local trail, and even getting a puppy to keep me active. Thanks to these healthy lifestyle modifications and daily blood pressure medication, I am now in control of my blood pressure.

MU/PD: You should be proud of yourself for managing your blood pressure. How did you become aware of lifestyle modifications?

Rolanda: I felt alone after receiving a diagnosis of high blood pressure and a heart attack. I didn't know many people who had gone through what I had with my health just now. So I started working as a volunteer for the American Heart Association (AHA), first at health fairs and later as a spokesman for the organization's Go Red for Women campaign on a national level. From there, I discovered WomenHeart, a nationwide group for women with heart disease. As a WomenHeart Champion, I currently co-lead a support group in Nashville, Tennessee, for women who have just received a heart disease diagnosis or have experienced cardiovascular events like heart attacks. I now broadcast a local radio show on women's concerns, including women's health, every fourth Sunday.

What guidance do you have for people who may have just received a high blood pressure diagnosis?

Rolanda: People must be aware of the sodium content of their food. I didn't realize that a big contributing cause was having too much sodium until I had my heart attack. Read the nutrition label and ingredients list before cleaning out the pantry and cabinets. Use a tiny salt shaker daily and fill it to the brim with salt if you're aiming to reduce your sodium intake rather than a table salt shaker. Additionally, learn how to season meals without adding salt by utilizing spices and herbs.

Diet and Nutritional Support for Blood Pressure Control

Nutrition and diet management of blood pressure is a crucial component of overall cardiovascular health. Here are some dietary recommendations to assist with controlling blood pressure. Some of these were already discussed. But I'll try to breeze through them once more.

- **Reduce Your Sodium Intake:** High sodium intake is closely associated with high blood pressure. If you have hypertension or are at risk, keep your daily sodium consumption to less than 2,300 mg, or even lower to 1,500 mg.

Steer clear of fast meals, canned soups, processed foods, and salty snacks. Instead, choose fresh, healthy ingredients, and flavor your dishes with herbs and spices.

- **Increase Your Potassium Intake**: Eating meals high in potassium can help reduce the impact of salt on your blood pressure. Bananas, oranges, avocados, spinach, sweet potatoes, tomatoes, and beans are all excellent suppliers of potassium. Aim for a daily potassium intake of 3,500–4,700 mg.
- **Consider adopting the DASH diet**: The Dietary Approaches to Stop Hypertension (DASH) diet is a well-known dietary strategy for controlling blood pressure. Lean proteins, whole grains, fruits, vegetables, and low-fat dairy products are highlighted. Additionally, it encourages cutting back on sodium intake and contains healthy fats like

those in nuts, seeds, and olive oil.

- Limit your intake of saturated and trans fats because they can elevate blood cholesterol levels and increase your chance of developing heart disease. Pick skinless fowl, fish, lentils, and low-fat dairy items as your lean protein sources. Instead of butter or lard, substitute healthier fats such olive oil, avocado oil, and canola oil.
- Eat more foods high in magnesium because this mineral helps to control blood pressure. Consume foods high in magnesium, such as leafy greens, nuts, seeds, whole grains, and legumes.
- **Watch Your Alcohol Intake:** Drinking too much alcohol might cause blood pressure to rise. Limit your alcohol intake to moderate levels, which for men and women equates to no more than two drinks per day.

- **Maintain a Healthy Weight**: If you are overweight, losing weight can greatly reduce your blood pressure. To reach and maintain a healthy weight, combine a balanced diet with frequent exercise.
- Watch your coffee intake because, while it doesn't affect blood pressure over the long run, it can spike it momentarily. Limit your consumption of coffee, tea, energy drinks, and soda if you are sensitive to caffeine.
- **Portion Control**: Eating too much might lead to weight gain and high blood pressure. Use smaller dishes and pay attention to portion sizes to reduce how much food you eat.
- **Be Wary of Added Sugars**: Consuming a lot of sugar has been linked to higher blood pressure. Limit your intake of sugar-sweetened foods and beverages and choose

healthy substitutes like whole fruits.

Remember to seek specialized dietary counsel from a medical expert or registered dietitian, especially if you have underlying medical issues or are taking drugs that could interact with certain foods.

Before we discuss the second aspect that contributes to the best possible functioning of cardiovascular health, one more point should be made.

High blood pressure does exist, but you can't see it, I assure you. Additionally, you frequently cannot feel it. The majority of hypertensive persons experience no symptoms.

But whether you're one of the 78 million Americans who have hypertension or one of the 70 million who have prehypertension (blood pressure readings beyond the recommended range), it's crucial to understand the effects it has on your health and to take steps right away to lower your readings.

A thorough strategy that combines dietary adjustments,

lifestyle changes, and, if necessary, medication procedures is needed to lower high blood pressure. You can drastically lower your blood pressure and lower your risk of heart disease and stroke by using the techniques described in this book. Adopting these new behaviors may take some time and work, but the rewards are well worth it. Keep in mind that high blood pressure is manageable, and that you can regulate your health with the correct resources and assistance. The most crucial thing is to stick with your new regimen and be committed to it. To live a better, happier life for years to come, start making little changes today.

2. heart wellness

Heart care is the process of protecting and improving the health of the heart and circulatory system. The heart pumps blood while simultaneously supplying the body with nutrition and oxygen. If you want to live a long and healthy life, you need to take care of your heart.

Heart care has many components, including dietary adjustments, therapeutic procedures, and preventative measures. It works to prevent and cure problems related to the heart, including as coronary artery disease, heart attacks, heart failure, arrhythmias, and valvular abnormalities.

Why is the heart's health crucial.

As was already said, the heart is a beautiful organ that is vital to sustaining life. It acts as the primary pump for the circulatory system, transporting oxygen-rich blood throughout the body and making sure that all organs and tissues have the nutrients they need to function optimally. Heart health is so crucial to overall wellbeing and lifespan that it is impossible to overstate its significance.

- **Prevention of heart disease:** Heart disease, which encompasses conditions including coronary artery disease, heart attacks, and heart failure, is a leading cause of death worldwide. By prioritizing their heart health, individuals can significantly reduce their risk of developing these debilitating conditions. Regular health exams, risk factor control, and healthy lifestyle choices are all preventive measures that can help find and fix issues before they worsen.

- **Improved Quality of Life:** People with healthy hearts can lead fulfilling lives filled with activity. When the heart is in good health, it can effectively distribute oxygenated blood to the muscles, organs, and tissues, ensuring that these structures receive an adequate supply of both nutrients and oxygen. As a result, people can engage in hobbies, daily activities, and exercise without becoming unduly exhausted or uncomfortable.

- **Longevity and Life Expectancy:** A longer life expectancy is closely correlated with maintaining good heart health. A heart-healthy lifestyle and effective risk factor management can help people live years longer. Maintaining cardiovascular health leads to a longer, healthier lifespan and reduces the possibility of acquiring potentially fatal cardiac conditions.

- **Prevention of Coexisting Conditions:** The management of a number of coexisting conditions has a direct impact on heart health. For instance, keeping blood pressure within healthy ranges reduces the risk of kidney illness and a stroke. Similar to how avoiding the buildup of plaque in the arteries through good cholesterol management can reduce the risk of heart attacks and strokes.

- **Positive Impact on Mental Health:** Strong links exist between mental and cardiovascular health.

Regular exercise and a balanced diet may help maintain a healthy heart, which has a positive effect on mental health and reduces the risk of depression and anxiety. Enhancing one's body image, self-confidence, and general wellbeing are also encouraged by adopting heart-healthy habits.

Along with economic and social advantages, promoting heart health has broader societal effects. By reducing the burden of heart disease, healthcare systems can better allocate resources and people can avoid costly medical treatments and long-term care associated to heart disorders. Additionally, having a healthy heart means that a person is more likely to be active and productive in both their personal and professional lives, which helps the economy and society as a whole.

Maintaining heart health is crucial for a number of reasons. In addition to delaying the beginning of potentially deadly diseases, a healthy heart also promotes general wellbeing, lengthens life, protects against coexisting diseases, and has positive effects on mental health. Emphasizing heart health through lifestyle modifications, regular checkups, and the right medical procedures can help people improve their well-being and lead richer, more active lives.

frequent maladies and conditions linked to the heart

It's important to remember that this is not a complete list and that there are other heart-related ailments and diseases in addition to the common heart-related conditions. Depending on the ailment, different causes, signs, tests, and therapies are available.

Here are a few common heart problems along with brief descriptions of each:

Coronary Artery Disease (CAD)

Coronary artery disease is brought on by plaque buildup in the arteries that supply the heart muscle with oxygen-rich blood. The plaque is composed of calcium, fat, cholesterol, and other substances. Over time, the plaque may harden, narrow the arteries, and lessen blood flow to the heart. This could have a number of effects, including angina (chest pain), heart attacks, and others.

2. A myocardial infarction or heart attack:

When blood flow to a section of the heart muscle is suddenly cut off, a heart attack occurs. Usually, this happens as a result of a blood clot forming on top of a plaque in a coronary artery. Due to a lack of blood and oxygen, the heart muscle may suffer long-term damage. Possible heart attack symptoms include chest pain or discomfort, shortness of breath, sweating, nausea, and lightheadedness. To prevent cardiac damage, it's critical to get medical attention very away.

3. heart illness

Heart failure is a condition where the heart is unable to pump enough blood to meet the body's demands. Numerous illnesses, including coronary artery disease, hypertension, injuries to the heart muscle, and problems with the heart valves, can cause it. There may be symptoms such as difficulty breathing, tiredness, fluid retention, swollen ankles or legs, and difficulty carrying out daily activities.

4. Heart arrhythmias

Arrhythmias, or irregular cardiac rhythms, are the result of disrupted electrical impulses that regulate the heart's beating. This can cause the heart to beat excessively quickly (tachycardia), too slowly (bradycardia), or irregularly. Although some arrhythmias are not harmful, others can. Typical symptoms include palpitations, a rapid heartbeat, dizziness, fainting, and discomfort in the chest.

5. Heart valve conditions

Heart valve diseases happen when the heart's internal blood flow control valves are damaged. Valve diseases can take many different shapes, including:

- **Aortic Stenosis:** Blood flow from the heart to the body's other organs is impeded when the aortic valve narrows.

- **Mitral Valve Prolapse**: If the mitral valve flaps do not completely shut, blood may leak backward into the left atrium.
- **Mitral Valve Stenosis**: Blood flow from the left atrium to the left ventricle is impeded as the mitral valve narrows.

The mitral valve doesn't shut tightly, allowing blood to seep back into the left atrium.

- Tricuspid Valve Regurgitation: Blood flows into the right atrium from the left side when the tricuspid valve does not shut tightly.

6. Congenital Heart Defects:

Congenital heart defects are structural anomalies that are present at birth and have an impact on the structure and operation of the heart. These defects could have an impact on the heart walls, heart valves, or blood vessels. The intensity and symptoms may range widely, from trivial occurrences that might not require treatment to complex issues that require surgical intervention.

7. Cardiomyopathy

Cardiomyopathies are illnesses that affect the heart muscle and make it more difficult for the heart to adequately pump blood. Dilated cardiomyopathy (heart chambers weaken and widen), hypertrophic cardiomyopathy (heart muscle thickens), and limited cardiomyopathy (heart muscle gets stronger) are just a few of the different types of cardiomyopathy. Symptoms include fatigue, shortness of breath, edema, and irregular heartbeats.

Heart health and lifestyle considerations

Lifestyle choices have a big impact on heart health. Here are some significant areas where your lifestyle may affect the health of your heart:

- **Diet and nutrition:** A healthy diet is essential to maintaining heart health. Eating a balanced diet rich in fruits, vegetables, whole grains, lean meats, and healthy fats can reduce the chance of developing heart disease. Because they elevate blood pressure, raise cholesterol levels, and encourage obesity, saturated and trans fats, cholesterol, sodium, and added sweets should all be ingested in moderation.

- **Physical Activity:** Regular physical activity is essential for a healthy heart. You can improve your cardiovascular fitness, maintain a healthy weight, and lower your blood pressure by engaging in moderate-intensity aerobic activity, such as brisk walking, running, swimming, or cycling, for at least 150 minutes each week.
- **Quit smoking:** Heart disease is made more likely by smoking. The benefits of quitting smoking and avoiding secondhand smoke on heart health are significant. Smoking damages blood arteries, reduces oxygen flow to tissues, raises the risk of atherosclerosis, and causes blood clots to form more frequently.

Quitting smoking improves heart and general health in the short and long terms.

- **Weight control:** Maintaining a healthy weight is crucial for heart health. Obesity and excess body weight have an impact on a number of heart-related risk factors, including high blood pressure, high cholesterol, insulin resistance, and inflammation. By adopting a balanced diet, engaging in regular exercise, and living a healthy lifestyle, people can reach and maintain a healthy weight and reduce their risk of heart disease.
- **Reduction of Stress:** Prolonged stress might be bad for your heart. Long-term stress may result in elevated blood pressure, an accelerated heartbeat, and unhealthy coping behaviors like binge eating, excessive alcohol consumption, or smoking. Although stress can be

harmful to the heart, it can be handled through relaxation techniques, consistent exercise, adequate sleep, and stress-relieving activities.

- Excessive alcohol use raises the risk of arrhythmias, heart failure, and excessive blood pressure. Health regulations recommend using alcohol in moderation. For men and women, up to two drinks per day are considered moderate amounts of alcohol use.

For the early detection and treatment of heart-related disorders, routine medical exams are essential. Regular tests, such as blood pressure readings, cholesterol checks, and diabetes testing, can help identify and treat potential risk factors and illnesses that may have an influence on heart health. Cooperation with healthcare specialists is essential for maintaining a close eye on and managing any current disorders.

heart function and anatomy

The heart is a muscular organ located in the chest cavity that circulates blood throughout the body. Its unique structure is a result of the four chambers, valves, and complicated blood artery network. Here is a list of its key components:

The chambers of the heart are as follows:

1. **Right Atrium:** The right atrium receives deoxygenated blood from the body through two large veins called the superior vena cava and inferior vena cava.

2. **Right Ventricle:** From the right atrium, the blood flows into the right ventricle, which then pumps the deoxygenated blood to the lungs for oxygenation.

3. **Left Atrium:** Oxygenated blood from the lungs enters the left atrium through the pulmonary veins.

4. **Left Ventricle:** The left atrium passes the oxygenated blood into the left ventricle, which is the

largest and strongest chamber. It pumps the oxygenated blood out to the rest of the body.

Valves of the Heart:

- The Heart's Valves The Tricuspid Valve prevents blood from returning to the right atrium while the heart contracts. It is located between the right atrium and right ventricle.

- The pulmonary valve, which is positioned between the right ventricle and the pulmonary artery, allows blood to go from the heart to the lungs but prevents blood flow back into the ventricle.

- The left atrium and left ventricle are separated by the mitral valve, which ensures that oxygenated blood only flows in one direction from the atrium to the ventricle and prevents backflow.

- Aortic Valve. The aortic valve, which is located between the left ventricle and the body's main artery, the aorta, permits blood to leave the heart while forbidding it from returning.

Blood Circulation: The heart works as a pump to transport blood throughout the body. Blood circulates in the body in a certain way:

- The superior and inferior vena cava transport deoxygenated blood from the body to the right atrium.
- When the right atrium contracts, blood is propelled through the tricuspid valve and into the right ventricle.
- The pulmonary valve allows deoxygenated blood to enter the pulmonary artery when the right ventricle contracts.
- The pulmonary artery carries the deoxygenated blood to the lungs, where it inhales oxygen and exhales carbon dioxide.
- Oxygenated blood is returned to the heart via the pulmonary veins and enters the left atrium.

- When the left atrium contracts, oxygen-rich blood is forced past the mitral valve and into the left ventricle.
- The left ventricle, which has the highest force of the three chambers, contracts and forces oxygenated blood past the aortic valve and into the aorta.
- An arterial network that further divides into capillaries and arterioles, smaller blood vessels, delivers oxygenated blood to all parts of the body.
- The capillaries collect waste and carbon dioxide while supplying tissues with oxygen and nutrients.

After returning to the heart through a network of veins, deoxygenated blood eventually reaches the superior and inferior vena cava, where the cycle is repeated.

Blood vessels and the circulatory system:

The three main types of blood vessels that make up the cardiovascular system are capillaries, veins, and arteries.

Arteries: Blood vessels that are both muscular and elastic, arteries carry oxygen-rich blood from the heart to the body's tissues. Because of their thick walls, they can endure the high pressure that heartbeats produce. When arteries branch out, the resulting smaller arterioles aid in further regulating blood flow into capillaries.

Capillaries: Capillaries are tiny, thin-walled blood veins that connect arterioles and venules. They act as the point of contact between the nearby tissues and the blood. Oxygen and nutrients diffuse from the capillaries into the tissues, whereas waste products and carbon dioxide diffuse from the tissues into the capillaries to be eliminated.

Veins: Veins transport deoxygenated blood away from the capillaries and back to the heart. They have thinner walls than arteries and valves that prevent blood from flowing backward. Veins gradually unite to produce larger channels that send deoxygenated blood to the right atrium of the heart, forming the superior and inferior vena cava.

Blood constantly circulates via this system of blood vessels, powered by the heart's pumping action. Veins return deoxygenated blood to the heart, and arteries carry oxygenated blood out from the heart, completing the circulatory cycle.

Overall, the intricate system of blood vessels and the heart's structure and operations ensure that nutrition, oxygen, and waste products are efficiently transported throughout the body, providing all organs and tissues with the support they require.

Heart disease prevention strategies

Before I go on, I want you to understand how important it is to consult your doctor in order to get advice and recommendations that are uniquely suited to your particular health situation.

Adopt a Healthful Diet: As part of a well-balanced and nutrient-rich diet, eat a variety of fruits, vegetables, whole grains, lean proteins (like fish and poultry), and healthy fats (like olive oil and avocados). Reduce your consumption of trans fats, saturated fatty acids, added sugars, cholesterol, sodium, and added sugars. Fatty fish, flaxseeds, and walnuts are examples of foods strong in omega-3 fatty acids, which are heart-healthy.

Regular Physical Activity: Aim for 150 minutes of moderate aerobic activity per week, or at least 75 minutes of vigorous aerobic activity. Jogging, brisk walking, swimming, cycling, and dancing are all fantastic possibilities. Include strength-training exercises as well to improve muscle strength and flexibility. Consult your healthcare provider before starting any new exercise program.

Keep Your Weight Healthy: Try to maintain a healthy weight that is appropriate for your height and body type. A person is more likely to develop heart disease if they are overweight, especially around the waist. Combine a nutritious diet with regular exercise for the best weight management results.

Steer clear of smoking and passive smoking: Smoking raises the risk of heart disease. Quitting smoking is the best thing you can do for your heart and general health. Avoid exposure to secondhand smoke as well because it may be harmful.

Only occasionally drink alcohol, and keep your consumption to a minimum. Moderation for women means no more than one drink per day, while for men it means no more than two. Abuse of alcohol can make people more susceptible to illnesses related to the heart, such as high blood pressure and heart failure.

Reduce Stress: Constant stress can make heart disease worse. Find pleasurable pastimes and hobbies as well as healthy stress-reduction techniques like yoga, meditation, and deep breathing exercises. You can also enlist the aid of close friends and family and maintain a healthy work-life balance.

Control Blood Pressure: High blood pressure, often known as hypertension, is a major risk factor for heart disease.

Regularly check your blood pressure and, if necessary, use prescription drugs to keep it within a reasonable range. You should also make lifestyle adjustments to reduce your sodium intake, adopt a balanced diet, keep a healthy weight, exercise frequently, and manage stress.

Manage Cholesterol Levels: High levels of LDL (the bad cholesterol) and low levels of HDL (the good cholesterol) can both cause atherosclerosis and heart disease. Adopt a heart-healthy diet, exercise frequently, avoid trans fats, and, if required, consult with your doctor to take medication to lower your cholesterol.

Control Diabetes: If you have diabetes, it's important to manage it well because uncontrolled diabetes increases your risk of heart disease. When it comes to regulating your blood sugar levels with medicine, food, exercise, and regular monitoring, follow your doctor's advise.

Get Regular Checkups: Schedule regular checkups with your doctor to monitor your heart's health. Your blood pressure may be taken, your cholesterol assessed, your risk for diabetes screened, among other tests, during these assessments. Early risk factor detection and management are essential to maintaining cardiovascular health.

Always remember to see your healthcare provider for advice and customized recommendations based on your current state of health. By implementing these preventive measures, you may significantly reduce your risk of getting heart disease and enhance your general cardiovascular health.

How the three women's heart ailments are managed.

By eating a heart-healthy diet, getting regular exercise, and managing your stress, you can prevent developing heart disease or cardiovascular disease. If you already have heart disease, these habits are even more important. The American Heart Association estimates that one in three women in the nation suffer from a cardiovascular disease. The good news is that you can still live a happy, healthy life despite a diagnosis.

Three women share their inspiring stories and offer guidance on how to deal with cardiac disease in this article.

1. Jen Hyde, a poet, teacher, wife, and author of books.

The way Jen Hyde looks completely conceals her cardiac issue. Her congenital heart issue, which she had had from birth, required surgery. In the 1980s, a lot of study was done on her condition, tetralogy of Fallot, but there was considerably less focus on diseases of the heart valves. Doctors warned Hyde's parents that she would become worse, but at this point, heart valve surgery was the best option.

Hyde, who was 25 at the time, learned that she would need a new heart valve in 2010. In addition, Hyde says, "I was finishing up my first year of graduate school, so it was really scary." I had planned to continue writing my book all summer.

The shock of the diagnosis was increased by the fact that Hyde had stopped obtaining regular care. Since she was an undergraduate at college, she had not seen a cardiologist. Finally, she managed to track down a cardiologist in New York. Hyde's two options for replacing a heart valve were a mechanical valve or a bioprosthetic valve (sometimes called tissue valves). Her doctor discussed the benefits, drawbacks, and probable health repercussions of each option. She decided to use the bioprosthetic valve because it did not necessitate long-term blood thinning medication use.

Hyde acknowledged that the majority of her early health knowledge came from her cardiologist. Later, she learned how helpful the American Heart Association's Patient Support Network was. Through the network, she found support from other patients, learned about recent studies, and received lists of questions to ask her doctors.

"I genuinely think it's a fantastic advantage that I have to think about my health frequently. I am more involved. I take my diet into account. I make better decisions, Hyde asserts.My physical endurance has substantially improved since my valve was replaced.

The fact that Jen will give birth to her first child in April 2018 makes all of this excellent news. Definitely a guy.

When asked what advice she would provide to women who are hesitant to visit the doctor, she offered three options.

(1) Think of your doctor as a confidante or "professional best friend for your heart."

(2) Request a second opinion without holding back.

(3) Ask a ton of questions.

2. Wife, advocate of women's health, friend, and volunteer Elizabeth Beard

Elizabeth Beard didn't initially understand she had heart disease; she had smoked for 35 years until giving it up in 2012 at the age of 52. She began a walking regimen at around the same time and soon began to experience tight calves and numbness in her feet.

She never connected her own health risk factors with heart disease despite having a family history of the condition. She initially assumed it had to do with the fact that she was obese and out of shape. Peripheral artery disease, or PAD, a cardiovascular illness where plaque builds up in the small vessels and prevents blood flow to a person's legs, feet, or arms, was discovered to be the cause of what she initially assumed to be a minor leg issue.

According to Beard, everything moved so swiftly that it took him only two weeks to go from receiving a diagnosis to having bypass surgery. My primary care physician initially diagnosed me, but at the time, I didn't receive much information regarding the illness.

In order to learn more about PAD, she started reading medical papers on her own.

Beard's surgeon and cardiologist cautioned her that if she delayed having bypass surgery, she might lose both of her legs and that she was at great danger of dying from a heart attack or stroke.

In the absence of physical therapy, akin to the cardiac rehab offered to patients following a heart attack or open heart surgery, Beard underwent her own rehabilitation with the help of her husband. Her rehabilitation progressed slowly and occasionally hurt. She experienced major blockages in her aorta and femoral arteries after the surgery, which made it impossible for her to get to her mailbox.

Since starting to do this roughly five years ago, Beard has increased his daily walking distance from a few feet to three to five miles. The standard treatment for PAD involves walking as far as you can before experiencing pain, and then attempting to go a little bit further.

Beard acknowledges that her experience with PAD had a good effect on her way of life, despite the fact that she would never wish a cardiovascular ailment on anyone. She constantly takes her medication, exercises frequently, and eats better—no more fried food. Since Beard was identified as having PAD, Medicare has authorized supervised exercise treatment, or SET, for PAD patients.

According to Beard, heart disease really is a "whole body disease," meaning that your mind and emotions have an affect on how you feel and that stress or depression will have an impact on your heart.

In the end, this will help in heart disease prevention. Investigate the root of the problem before implementing a heart-healthy lifestyle.

3. **Stephanie Lang is a mother, a wife, and a physical therapy assistant who likes to exercise.**

Stephanie was in fantastic health and had reduced 60 pounds before learning she had heart problems. She had nausea and dizziness one day while exercising at the gym, and she eventually passed out. She originally resisted going to the hospital, but after complying, she learned she had spontaneous coronary artery dissection, which led to a heart attack.

Lang also underwent cardiac rehabilitation, which involved weekly group sessions and daily individual sessions. "It was quite challenging at first. I got three stents, and I still had a lot to learn about my diagnosis," Lang remembers.

In the group meetings, we talked about food, handling emotions, and managing stress because stress boosts blood pressure.

With the support of MyFitnessPal, a Fitbit she wears every day to log her steps, six days a week of exercise, and a chest strap called MyZone that enables her to keep her heart rate in a healthy range when she exercises at the gym, Lang is doing well today.

She lives a similar healthy lifestyle to the Lang family: "The kids don't always like it, but generally speaking there's no soda in the house. We consume a lot of vegetables, poultry, and turkey. A red meat ban.

She urges all women to speak up for themselves and ask questions, mentioning situations in which medications may be provided as part of regular practice and highlighting the significance of learning why they are a good option for you.

Lang suggests being aware of your statistics, getting regular checkups, and not being reluctant to see a doctor if anything doesn't feel right.

3. CHOLESTEROL CONTENT

Before I go into great depth about what cholesterol is, keep in mind that it is not inherently bad because our bodies require it to operate properly. Maintaining equilibrium between the various kinds of cholesterol and keeping them within a healthy range is the key to promoting heart health.

What is cholesterol, exactly? kinds, underlying causes, and consequences for human health.

Cholesterol is a substance that naturally occurs in our bodies and is crucial for maintaining our overall health. This waxy, fatty substance, which is also present in some of the foods we eat, is present in every cell. Despite the fact that cholesterol has a reputation for having bad effects, it's important to understand that our bodies need cholesterol to function properly. We'll examine the effects of cholesterol on our health in this topic, as well as its applications and various types.

Cholesterol serves a number of important functions in our bodies. It is a crucial component of cell membranes that gives cells their fluidity and stability. It also contributes to the production of hormones including estrogen, progesterone, and testosterone, which regulate a variety of biological processes. Additionally, cholesterol is a precursor to vitamin D, which is essential for maintaining bone health, and it helps to create bile acids, which facilitate the digestion of fats.

Our bodies may produce cholesterol on their own, primarily in the liver, but it can also be obtained from diet. Cholesterol is a nutrient that is only present in meals derived from animals, such as meat, poultry, eggs, and dairy products. It's important to keep in mind that dietary cholesterol has less of an impact on blood cholesterol levels than saturated and trans fats, which can raise LDL cholesterol.

When discussing cholesterol, the terms low-density lipoprotein (LDL) and high-density lipoprotein (HDL) cholesterol are frequently employed.

Since it can contribute to the development of artery plaque, LDL cholesterol is usually referred to as "bad" cholesterol. When there is too much LDL cholesterol in the circulation, it can accumulate on the artery walls and lead to atherosclerosis. Atherosclerosis, or the hardening and constriction of the arteries, raises the risk of heart disease and stroke.

HDL cholesterol, on the other hand, is referred to as "good" cholesterol. Extra cholesterol from the bloodstream is transported by the HDL molecule to the liver, where it can be broken down and expelled from the body. Higher HDL cholesterol levels are associated with a decreased risk of heart disease.

Maintaining healthy levels of LDL and HDL cholesterol is essential for cardiovascular health. Having high levels of LDL cholesterol can increase your risk of developing heart disease along with other risk factors including smoking, having diabetes, or having high blood pressure. On the other hand, higher HDL cholesterol levels are normally seen favorably because they can help with heart disease prevention.

When discussing cholesterol levels, medical professionals typically mention LDL cholesterol as a crucial indicator of cardiovascular health. Depending on the person's risk factors, normal LDL cholesterol targets range from below 100 mg/dL to beyond 200 mg/dL. LDL cholesterol levels can be reduced by altering one's lifestyle, such as by giving up smoking, adopting a nutritious diet, and engaging in regular exercise.

Medication may be advised if dietary and lifestyle changes are insufficient to control cholesterol levels. Statins are a class of medications frequently used to lower LDL cholesterol. They work by halting a liver enzyme's ability to produce cholesterol. Other medications, such fibrates and niacin, can aid in raising HDL cholesterol levels or lowering triglyceride levels, another type of blood fat.

A person's blood cholesterol levels must be regularly checked in order to assess their risk of heart disease and to guide treatment decisions. To determine the best course of action given the variety of treatment options, it is essential to speak with medical experts.

In conclusion, cholesterol performs a number of biological activities in our bodies, including the manufacturing of hormones, the building of cell membranes, and digestion. However, cardiovascular diseases can develop as a result of abnormally high LDL cholesterol. A comprehensive cholesterol control strategy that also promotes overall heart health includes changing one's lifestyle, taking medication as needed, and routine monitoring.

CHAPTER 3:

METABOLIC HEALTH.
The word **"metabolic health"** refers to the overall state of our body's metabolism, which involves a number of chemical processes that occur inside our cells to convert food into energy. Among the many factors it takes into account are insulin sensitivity, blood sugar control, lipid (fat) metabolism, and total energy balance. When our metabolic health is at its greatest, these processes function well, enhancing general wellness and reducing the risk of metabolic diseases including obesity, type 2 diabetes, and cardiovascular diseases.

Metabolic health is crucial since it is necessary to maintaining our overall health and wellbeing. Major explanations for the importance of metabolic health include the following:

Weight management: A healthy metabolism aids in maintaining a healthy body weight by efficiently utilizing the calories from food. A robust metabolism helps to maintain a healthy weight by burning calories for energy effectively. A slow metabolism, however, can lead to weight gain and obesity, which are connected to a number of health problems like diabetes, heart disease, and joint problems.

Blood Sugar Control: Maintaining a healthy metabolism helps with blood sugar management. When we eat carbohydrates, they are transformed into glucose, which is then transported to our cells and used as an energy source. Insulin, a pancreatic hormone, plays a vital role in controlling blood sugar levels. In those with healthy metabolisms, insulin effectively facilitates glucose uptake by cells. Although insulin resistance, which occurs when cells lose their receptivity to insulin and blood sugar levels rise, can be brought on by deteriorating metabolic health, it also increases the risk of type 2 diabetes.

Lipid Metabolism and Heart Health: The state of our metabolic health determines how well our bodies can process lipids and cholesterol. A healthy metabolism helps to regulate blood lipid levels and maintains the balance between "good" cholesterol (HDL) and "bad" cholesterol (LDL) in the blood. An optimum lipid profile, which contains higher levels of HDL cholesterol and lower levels of LDL cholesterol, is associated with a lower risk of cardiovascular diseases, such as heart attacks and strokes. On the other side, an unbalanced lipid profile brought on by poor metabolic health might cause the arteries to produce plaque, which can constrict them and lessen blood flow.

Energy and vitality: Food is efficiently converted into energy by a healthy metabolism, providing the fuel needed for everyday activities and the best possible operation of bodily functions. We feel energized, awake, and capable of successfully completing both physical and mental tasks when our metabolism is working at its best. Poor metabolic health, on the other hand, might result in weariness, lethargy, and decreased productivity.

Lifespan and Long-Term Health: There is a close connection between metabolic health and long-term health consequences. Diabetes and obesity, two chronic metabolic diseases, increase the risk of a variety of disorders, including cardiovascular disease, kidney disease, nerve damage, and many cancers. We can reduce our chance of developing chronic diseases, possibly even live longer, and live happier, more fulfilling lives by improving our metabolic health.

The state of one's metabolism can be influenced by a number of variables, including genetics, nutrition, physical activity, sleep patterns, stress levels, and environmental influences. By living a healthy lifestyle that includes eating a balanced diet, working out frequently, lowering stress, and getting enough sleep, the risk of metabolic illnesses can be significantly reduced.

In conclusion, it is crucial for overall health to maintain metabolic health. It affects blood sugar control, weight management, lipid metabolism, energy levels, and long-term health impacts. By putting metabolic health first and increasing it through food and lifestyle choices, we may increase our quality of life, reduce our risk of developing chronic diseases, and perhaps even extend our lifetime.

How can having improved metabolic health lead to living a longer, healthier life?

Improving metabolic health can have a big impact on both lengthening lifespan and promoting general health and wellbeing. Improving metabolic health can assist living a longer, healthier life in the following key ways:

1. **Decreased Risk of Chronic Diseases:** A few of the chronic conditions that are closely linked to poor metabolic health include obesity, type 2 diabetes, cardiovascular disease, and certain types of cancer. By improving your metabolic health, you can significantly lower

your risk of developing these issues. For instance, maintaining a healthy weight, managing blood sugar levels, and enhancing lipid profiles may reduce the chance of developing heart disease, diabetes, and obesity, which are the main causes of premature death.

Heart health can be improved since metabolic and cardiovascular health are interrelated. By managing your blood pressure, blood sugar, and cholesterol levels, you can significantly reduce your risk of developing heart disease, suffering a heart attack, or suffering a stroke. A healthy metabolism encourages higher levels of HDL cholesterol and lower levels of LDL cholesterol, both of which are essential for heart health.

Enhanced Energy and Vitality: By enhancing metabolic health, your body's mechanisms for producing and utilizing energy are improved. Your metabolism effectively converts food into energy when it's functioning at its peak, giving you the vigor you need to carry out daily tasks and physical exercise. This increased energy may have a good effect on your quality of life by enabling you to be more active, productive, and involved in many areas of your life.

Weight control: Maintaining a healthy weight is essential for metabolic health. By enhancing your metabolism, you may help your body be better able to suppress appetite, burn calories, and utilize nutrients. The ability to achieve and maintain a healthy weight has a direct impact on one's overall health and longevity.

Improved Cognitive Function: According to study, metabolism and brain health are closely related. Poor metabolic health, including insulin resistance and high blood sugar levels, has been related to cognitive decline and an increased risk of disorders like Alzheimer's disease. By improving your metabolic health, you may be able to support improved cognitive performance and reduce your risk of neurodegenerative diseases.

Reduced Inflammation and Chronic Oxidative Stress: Chronic inflammation and oxidative stress are the main causes of many diseases, including metabolic disorders. Improved cellular health and a decreased risk of acquiring chronic diseases are both promoted by improving metabolic health, which reduces oxidative stress and inflammation in the body.

Enhanced Longevity: By improving your metabolic health, you can have a positive effect on a variety of factors that affect longevity. Maintaining a healthy weight, managing blood sugar levels, enhancing lipid profiles, and reducing the risk of chronic diseases are all associated with living longer. A healthy metabolism encourages cellular activity and general wellbeing, which can result in a longer, more fulfilling life.

It's important to keep in mind that improving metabolic health requires a comprehensive approach. This comprises making appropriate dietary selections, getting regular exercise, managing stress, getting enough sleep, and avoiding unhealthy behaviors like smoking. Your ability to maximize your metabolic health for a longer, healthier life can be helped by working with medical professionals, nutritionists, and exercise specialists who can offer guidance tailored to your particular needs.

How does the metabolism work? It is what?

A wide variety of chemical processes that take place inside living things to support life are referred to as metabolism. It involves a series of metabolic reactions that convert food into energy, produce the chemicals needed for growth and repair, and eliminate waste. The metabolism has two main mechanisms:

1. **Catabolism**: This process involves breaking down complex molecules, such as carbohydrates, proteins, and fats, into smaller units to release energy. During catabolism, large

molecules are broken down through various reactions, such as digestion, to produce energy-rich molecules like adenosine triphosphate (ATP). ATP is the primary energy currency of cells and is used for various cellular functions.

2. **Anabolism**: The creation of complex molecules from simpler ones using the energy produced by catabolic reactions. Anabolic processes produce proteins, nucleic acids, and other materials so that cells and tissues can expand, mend, and sustain themselves.

The metabolic process relies on an intricate network of internal enzyme reactions and pathways. Here is a quick rundown of how metabolism works:

When we eat, food is mechanically and chemically digested in the gastrointestinal tract. Lipids transform into fatty acids, carbohydrates into simple sugars (like glucose), and proteins into amino acids. These smaller molecules can then enter the bloodstream thanks to the stomach lining. Here's a simplified overview of how metabolism works:

Cellular Uptake and Utilization: These substances are transported to all of the body's cells for usage after ingestion. For instance, insulin facilitates the entry of glucose into cells where it is used in the glycolysis process, which breaks down the sugar to produce ATP and other molecules. As they enter cells, amino acids and fatty acids can either be used immediately or stored for later use.

Energy Production: The breakdown of glucose and fatty acids takes place within mitochondria, which are cellular structures. Fatty acids and glucose are further broken down to produce ATP during cellular respiration. This process includes two chemical reactions that occur in the mitochondria: the Krebs cycle and oxidative phosphorylation.

Anabolic Reactions: Anabolic reactions use the energy produced by catabolic reactions to create complex compounds. Using amino acids to build proteins, nucleotides to create DNA and RNA, and the conversion of glucose molecules to glycogen for storage in the liver and muscles are just a few examples.

The metabolism is regulated by a sophisticated network of hormones, enzymes, and signaling molecules. Hormones like insulin and glucagon aid in blood sugar regulation in addition to regulating the storage and release of energy reserves. Enzymes act as catalysts, accelerating the chemical reactions involved in the metabolic process.

It's important to keep in mind that metabolism is a dynamic process that is influenced by factors including genetics, age, body composition, nutrition, exercise, and general health. By understanding how the metabolism works and making educated decisions about their diet, exercise program, and lifestyle, people may maintain a healthy and efficient metabolism.

The Connection between Metabolic Health and Lifespan Reduced Risk of Chronic Diseases: Chronic conditions that are closely associated with poor metabolic health include obesity, type 2 diabetes, cardiovascular disease, several types of cancer, and neurological diseases. By enhancing their metabolic health, people can significantly lower their risk of developing certain diseases, which may result in a longer lifespan.

Weight control: Maintaining a healthy weight necessitates consideration of metabolic health. Obesity, a condition characterized by excessive body fat, reduces life expectancy and raises the risk of contracting several chronic diseases. By enhancing metabolic health through healthy eating, regular exercise, and lifestyle choices, people can effectively manage their weight and reduce their risk of obesity-related health problems.

Control of Blood Sugar: Maintaining a healthy metabolism helps with blood sugar regulation. Conditions like insulin resistance and type 2 diabetes, which have compromised blood sugar management, are associated with an elevated risk of cardiovascular diseases and early mortality. By increasing their metabolic health, individuals can control their blood sugar levels, raise their insulin sensitivity, reduce their risk of developing diabetes-related complications, and improve their general health.

Cardiovascular health and metabolic health are closely linked. People with high blood pressure, dyslipidemia (an unbalanced lipid profile), and atherosclerosis (plaque growth in the arteries), which can also shorten lifespan, are more likely to develop cardiovascular disorders. By enhancing their metabolic health, people can reduce their chance of developing heart disease and its complications, control their blood pressure, and enhance their lipid profiles.

Reduced Inflammation and Oxidative Stress: The body's oxidative stress and inflammation are linked to poor metabolic health, which can expedite aging and lead to the emergence of chronic diseases. People can reduce oxidative stress and inflammation, which will enhance cellular health and length of life, by leading healthy lifestyles that enhance metabolic health.

Hormone balance: Hormones play a crucial role in metabolism and overall health. Thyroid, cortisol, and insulin hormonal abnormalities can affect metabolism and increase the risk of metabolic disorders. By maintaining hormonal balance through a healthy lifestyle and lowering stress levels, individuals can support good metabolic health and potentially increase their lifespan.

Cellular function is impacted by metabolic health, which also has an impact on how quickly people age. Maintaining cellular health and lifetime requires effective mitochondrial activity, DNA repair mechanisms, and efficient cellular functions. By improving their metabolic health, people may be able to promote healthier cellular aging and slow down the aging process.

illnesses influenced by metabolic disorders

Metabolic anomalies can lead to a variety of diseases and health problems. As examples, consider the following ailments connected to metabolic disorders:

A condition known as obesity is characterized by an abnormal accumulation of bodily fat. It frequently co-exists with metabolic illnesses such insulin resistance, dyslipidemia, and hypertension. Obesity increases the likelihood that people will develop type 2 diabetes, cardiovascular disease, certain cancers, sleep apnea, osteoarthritis, and fatty liver disease, to name a few.

Type 2 Diabetes: Type 2 diabetes is a metabolic disorder characterized by insulin resistance and elevated blood sugar levels. It occurs when the body's response to insulin declines or when insufficient amounts of insulin are created to effectively manage blood sugar. Type 2 diabetes increases the risk of cardiovascular disease, renal disease, nerve damage (neuropathy), eye problems (retinopathy), and foot problems.

Cardiovascular diseases: Metabolic conditions such obesity, insulin resistance, dyslipidemia, and hypertension affect the development of cardiovascular diseases. These conditions include heart attacks, strokes, peripheral artery disease, coronary artery disease, heart failure, and heart attacks. The effects of metabolic diseases include increased risk of blood clots, reduced blood flow, and plaque formation in the arteries.

Non-alcoholic Fatty Liver Disease (NAFLD): NAFLD is a condition that results in an accumulation of fat in the liver but is unrelated to excessive alcohol consumption. It significantly correlates with metabolic illnesses such obesity, insulin resistance, and dyslipidemia. NAFLD can progress into non-alcoholic steatohepatitis (NASH), cirrhosis, liver fibrosis, and liver cancer.

PCOS, or polycystic ovary syndrome, is a hormonal disorder

that mostly affects women and is associated with changes in metabolism. Polycystic ovaries, profuse hair growth, and irregular menstrual cycles are its defining features. The common side effects of PCOS include insulin resistance, obesity, dyslipidemia, and an increased risk of type 2 diabetes and cardiovascular diseases.

The metabolic syndrome is a group of co-occurring metabolic illnesses that includes central obesity, high blood pressure, high blood sugar, abnormal lipid profiles, and insulin resistance. People with metabolic syndrome are more prone to develop type 2 diabetes, heart disease, and stroke.

Gout: Gout is a severe form of arthritis that results in significant joint pain, swelling, and redness. It is brought on by the buildup of uric acid crystals in the joints. Elevated levels of uric acid in the blood, which can be brought on by metabolic issues like obesity, insulin resistance, and dyslipidemia, can lead to gout.

Alzheimer's disease: Research has linked metabolic problems, insulin resistance, and an increased risk of developing Alzheimer's and other forms of dementia. Although the precise mechanisms are still being studied, chronic inflammation, oxidative stress, and altered glucose metabolism in the brain are considered to play a part in the connection between metabolic abnormalities and cognitive decline.

These are just a few conditions where metabolic issues have been related to disease. It's important to stress that there may be complex and varied relationships between these illnesses and metabolic problems.

How to control or lessen them

In order to prevent and manage metabolic illnesses, a comprehensive strategy emphasizing dietary adjustments, medical therapies, and regular monitoring is needed. Metabolic diseases can be prevented and treated using the following methods:

- Consume a diet that is balanced and nutrient-dense by including a variety of fruits, vegetables, whole grains, lean meats, and healthy fats. Limit your intake of processed foods, sugary beverages, saturated fats, and sodium. Consider speaking with a licensed nutritionist for personalized nutritional guidance.

- Weight management: If you are overweight or obese, strive to reduce your calorie intake, eat smaller amounts, and engage in regular exercise to reach and maintain a healthy weight. With moderate and sustained weight loss, blood sugar levels, blood pressure, and lipid profiles are a few metabolic health indicators that can be addressed.

- Regular physical activity and exercise can help you manage your weight, enhance your cardiovascular health, and make insulin more sensitive. Attempt to complete at least 150 minutes of weight training and cardiovascular activity (such as cycling, jogging, or walking) each week.

- Medication and Medical Management: Several metabolic disorders, including type 2 diabetes, hypertension, and dyslipidemia, have symptoms that can be treated and managed with medication by medical professionals. It's essential to follow suggested treatment regimens and arrange regular exams.

- Blood Sugar Monitoring: Those who have diabetes or prediabetes must regularly test their blood sugar levels. It is now simpler to understand how variables like nutrition, activity, and medication may affect blood sugar levels. Speak with a healthcare professional for suggestions on monitoring frequency and objectives.

- Stress management: Prolonged stress might be detrimental to metabolic health. Practice stress-reduction techniques like yoga, deep breathing exercises, and mindfulness meditation, or engage in relaxing hobbies and diversions. Getting enough sleep is important for stress management and for maintaining overall health.

- Avoid Smoking: Smoking increases your risk of developing metabolic and cardiovascular issues. Ask for help and resources to quit smoking because doing so can improve your general health.

- Keep track of metabolic health indicators like body weight, blood pressure, and lipid profiles by scheduling routine health examinations. This facilitates early detection of changes or anomalies, allowing management and intervention as necessary.

- Education and Support: Research registered dietitians, medical authorities, and support groups that concentrate on metabolic disorders for information and assistance. Through knowledge and understanding, people can be empowered to make moral decisions and successfully manage their condition.

Keep in mind that everyone's journey to metabolic health is distinct, and that creating a tailored plan to prevent and treat metabolic disorders necessitates close coordination with healthcare professionals. Making long-term lifestyle alterations and consistently following medical advice can have a positive impact on metabolic health and general wellbeing.

You can significantly increase your life expectancy by adhering to the principles of metabolic health by making small, doable changes. Using the methods outlined in this book, you may take control of your metabolic health and set the stage for a longer, healthier life. Remember that a series of consistent, wise choices over time can make a significant difference.

Each simple action you take, such as selecting healthier foods, obtaining regular exercise, controlling stress, or seeking the appropriate medical guidance, will contribute to the optimization of your metabolic health. By focusing on these small actions, you can lengthen your life and achieve extraordinary outcomes.

The key is to embark on your quest for improved metabolic health with patience, persistence, and a growth mindset. No matter how little advancement you make, be conscious of it and celebrate each success as it occurs. Remember that even the slightest advancements matter when it comes to improving your health and prolonging your life.

Consider surrounding yourself with a group that is supportive and shares your goals when you first start down your route. Building a network of individuals committed to improving their metabolic health and with comparable goals can provide support, accountability, and a sense of belonging.

By living by the adage "Small Steps, Great Gain," you are investing in yourself and placing a high value on your long-term wellbeing. Your metabolic health will significantly improve over time as a result of the small changes you make now, potentially adding years to your life.

So, take that initial baby step today and let it be the catalyst for alterations that will change your life. You'll be appreciative of yourself later on when you enjoy the advantages of improved metabolic health, increased vigor, and a longer, healthier, and more fulfilling life.

CHAPTER 4

Respiratory health

I've always been a person who likes to be busy and socialize a lot. But everything changed when I was told I had a chronic respiratory illness, which rocked my world. All of a sudden, simply taking a breath was an effort, and even the smallest activities seemed like enormous undertakings.

I still clearly recall the day my doctor told me the bad news. I had gone in for a usual check-up on a lovely afternoon. I had no idea that my life was about to change dramatically. I was completely unprepared for the diagnosis, which left me feeling anxious about the future.

Every breath I took was important because I had a respiratory problem. Simple things like playing with my kids or climbing stairs became difficult undertakings that left me gasping for air and angry at my limitations. The persistent wheezing, pressure in my chest, and coughing have turned into unwelcome company that follows me day and night.

My respiratory health took center stage in my life, guiding my decisions and affecting the people I interacted with. I had to make changes and sacrifices I never thought I would have to make. I admired the freedom I once had as I watched friends

and relatives engage in activities
that were now out of my league.
But despite the difficulties and
setbacks, I discovered the real
significance of respiratory health.
It became clear that everything
else in life was pointless without
having sound lungs. I learned to
value the little periods of relief
when I could breathe fully and
profoundly without being
constrained. I came to understand
that maintaining my respiratory
system wasn't simply necessary
for survival; it was also the key
to take back my life.
I learned that making modest
changes could have a big impact
on lung health through
significant research, professional
consultations, and my own
experience with trial and error. I
experimented with breathing
techniques, made deliberate
lifestyle modifications, and
looked for the most effective
management techniques for my
illness.
I started to see improvements
over time. My energy levels rose
and my breathing became easier.
My sense of independence and
my capacity to engage in

activities that made me happy started to return. I felt the enormous effect that greater respiratory health had on my overall wellbeing with every modest step I took in that direction.

The value of respiratory health and the ability to make positive adjustments, no matter how tiny they may appear, were two things that this journey taught me. It motivated me to share my experience and the information I learned with others who might be dealing with comparable problems or looking for solutions to improve their respiratory health.

I want to provide you a thorough overview of respiratory health in this book's chapter. Together, we'll examine the peculiarities of the respiratory system, identify the prevalent illnesses that affect it, and delve into the dietary and exercise regimens that can help you achieve optimal lung function.

We may extend our lives and realize our full potential by arming ourselves with knowledge and making proactive moves toward better respiratory health. Together, let's begin this adventure, one breath at a time.

Why is respiratory health crucial for overall wellbeing

The importance of respiratory health goes well beyond just being able to breathe. Our ability to breathe is crucial to preserving our general health and quality of life. It facilitates the evacuation of waste products like carbon dioxide and acts as a doorway for oxygen, the life-sustaining gas that powers every cell in our bodies.

When our respiratory system performs at its best, it makes sure that our organs get a constant supply of oxygen, allowing them to work effectively. This process influences our mental and emotional health in addition to supporting physical activities. Here are some reasons why maintaining good respiratory health is crucial to our general health:

- **Vitality and Oxygenation:** Each cell in our body needs enough oxygen to be healthy and function properly. Oxygen powers cellular metabolism, giving different physiological processes energy. When our respiratory system is functioning properly, oxygen is effectively delivered to our tissues, enhancing vigor, endurance, and general physical performance.

- **Mental Acuity and Cognitive Function:** The brain depends heavily on a steady flow of oxygen to maintain peak performance. Reduced oxygen delivery to the brain caused by poor respiratory health can result in cognitive decline, attention deficit disorder, and memory issues. We improve mental acuity, concentration, and general cognitive performance by maintaining a healthy respiratory system.

- **Energy Levels and Fatigue Reduction:** A healthy respiratory system allows efficient oxygen exchange, which enables proper nutrition digestion and the creation of energy within our cells. We have more energy, feel less tired, and have better endurance when we get enough oxygen. Our ability to breathe comfortably during the day directly affects how energetic and productive we are.

- **Support for the immune system:** The respiratory system serves as a defensive mechanism, removing germs, allergens, and dangerous particles from the air we breathe. In addition to raising the risk of respiratory infections, a weakened immune system can also result from a compromised respiratory system. By preserving good respiratory health, we strengthen our immune system's capacity to fend off infections and sustain general health.
- Breathing exercises and methods, such as deep

diaphragmatic breathing, have a significant positive effect on our emotional balance and stress reduction. The body's relaxation response is triggered by deep, controlled breathing, which lowers tension and anxiety and fosters a sensation of peace. It functions as a potent self-regulation mechanism, enabling us to control our emotions and keep a healthy emotional balance.

- **lifespan and Quality of Life:** Enhanced lifespan and enhanced quality of life are directly correlated with optimal respiratory health. We can lower our chance of developing respiratory conditions like asthma and chronic obstructive pulmonary disease (COPD) by taking care of our lungs and boosting respiratory health. A longer, healthier life is ultimately the result of having good lungs, which also improve cardiovascular health and reduce the risk of related diseases.

Learning About the Respiratory System

The extraordinary network of tissues, organs, and structures that makes up the respiratory system enables the exchange of gases between our bodies and the environment. We can inhale the oxygen required for life and exhale carbon dioxide, a byproduct of cellular metabolism, thanks to it.

The lungs are two spongy, cone-shaped organs that are at the center of the respiratory system. They are situated in the chest cavity. The mediastinum, a central chamber that houses the heart, main blood arteries, and other crucial tissues, separates and protects the lungs from the ribcage.

When we breathe in air through our mouth or nose, the process of respiration starts. The trachea, also referred to as the windpipe, is where the air enters the body after passing through the throat and nasal passages or oral cavity. The trachea is a tubular structure made of cartilage rings that keeps it from collapsing and keeps the airway open.

The trachea splits into two major bronchi, one for each lung, inside the chest cavity. The bronchial tree is a complex network of branching airways formed by the subsequent division of the bronchi into smaller bronchial tubes. The bronchial tubes continue to separate into bronchioles, which are smaller and narrower tubes that eventually lead to alveoli, which are tiny air sacs.

The respiratory system's functional units, the alveoli, are where gases from the air and the bloodstream are exchanged. A network of capillaries surrounds these air sacs, allowing for the diffusion of oxygen into the circulation and the release of carbon dioxide into the alveoli for elimination.

The respiratory system depends on a variety of muscle activities to help flow air into and out of the lungs. A key component of breathing is the diaphragm, a dome-shaped muscle at the base of the lungs. The diaphragm flattens and contracts during inhalation, widening the chest cavity and generating a negative pressure that pulls air into the lungs. The diaphragm relaxes during exhale, allowing the lungs to contract and release carbon dioxide.

Other biological systems, especially the cardiovascular system, cooperate with the respiratory system. The heart then distributes the oxygen-rich blood to all the body's tissues and organs once it leaves the lungs. Deoxygenated blood that is also loaded with carbon dioxide is transported back to the lungs for removal at the same time. Understanding the respiratory system's intricate workings enables us to recognize its astonishing effectiveness and the crucial part it plays in maintaining life. Every stage of the process—from air inhalation through the mouth or nose to the exchange of gases within the alveoli—is meticulously planned to guarantee a constant flow of oxygen and the elimination of waste materials.

**respiratory system physiology
and anatomy**

The respiratory system is made
up of a number of related organs
and parts that cooperate to enable
the exchange of gases. The
following are some of the
respiratory system's crucial parts:
Air enters the respiratory system
through the nose, which is lined
with mucous membranes and
tiny hairs known as cilia.
Incoming air is filtered, warmed,
and moistened with the aid of the
nasal cavity.

- **Pharynx:** The pharynx,
  often known as the throat,
  is a muscular tube that
  joins the larynx to the
  nasal cavity and mouth. It
  acts as a conduit for food
  and air.
- **Larynx:** The larynx, also
  referred to as the voice
  box, houses the vocal
  cords and is where sound
  is produced. Additionally,
  it serves as a valve to keep
  food and liquids from
  getting into the respiratory
  system.
- **The trachea,** often known
  as the windpipe, is a stiff

tube made of cartilage
rings. It permits air to
enter the lungs and joins
the larynx to the bronchi.
The trachea separates into two
major bronchi, one for each lung,
creating the bronchi and
bronchial tree. The bronchial tree
is created inside the lungs as the
bronchi further split into smaller
bronchial tubes. The bronchial
tubes continue to branch into
bronchioles, which are
comparatively small and
narrower tubes.

- **Lungs:** Situated in the
  chest cavity, the lungs are
  a pair of cone-shaped
  organs. The ribcage
  encloses them, and the
  pleura, a slender
  membrane, serves as
  protection. To
  accommodate the area
  taken up by the heart, the
  right lung contains three
  lobes and the left lung
  only has two.
- **Alveoli:** The termini of the
  bronchioles are tiny air
  sacs referred to as alveoli.
  During gas exchange,
  oxygen diffuses into the

bloodstream and carbon dioxide is expelled from the bloodstream for elimination in these grape-like structures.

Ventilation and gas exchange are the respiratory system's two main tasks, according to respiratory system physiology.

- **Ventilation:** The act of breathing, which involves the passage of air into and out of the lungs, is referred to as ventilation. Inspiration and expiry make up its two stages. The chest cavity widens during inspiration as a result of the diaphragm and intercostal muscles contracting, creating a negative pressure that pulls air into the lungs. The diaphragm and intercostal muscles loosen up during expiration, allowing the lungs to recoil and evacuate air.

Gas Exchange: The alveoli are where gas exchange takes place. Inhaled air's oxygen diffuses past the alveolar walls and into the vicinity's capillaries, where it binds to hemoglobin in red blood cells. As carbon dioxide diffuses from capillaries into the alveoli to be exhaled, it is a waste product of cellular metabolism. The difference in partial pressures of oxygen and carbon dioxide between the air in the alveoli and the blood in the capillaries is what causes the exchange of gases. The heart then pumps the oxygenated blood to the body's tissues and organs after it has been carried. Deoxygenated blood, which is high in carbon dioxide, then returns to the lungs for gas exchange before being expelled during expiration.

The balance of oxygen and carbon dioxide in the body is maintained by the intricate interaction of chemical and neurological mechanisms that control the respiratory system. Through feedback systems involving the brain, respiratory centers, and chemoreceptors, variables such blood pH, carbon dioxide concentrations, and oxygen levels affect breathing rate and depth.

Understanding the respiratory system's anatomy and physiology helps us to understand the complex mechanisms that permit effective gas exchange and oxygenation of our bodies. We can promote our respiratory systems' optimal performance and ensure our bodies' general health by choosing healthy lifestyles and taking the necessary care of them.

How the respiratory system interacts with other systems in the body.

The respiratory system collaborates closely with a number of other body systems to guarantee effective gas exchange, preserve homeostasis, and promote general health. The respiratory system interacts with other systems in the following key ways:

- **Cardiovascular System:** The cardiovascular system and the respiratory system are interconnected. The circulatory system distributes these gases to and from bodily tissues, while the respiratory system delivers oxygen to

the bloodstream and
eliminates carbon dioxide.
The pulmonary veins carry
oxygen-rich blood from
the lungs to the left side of
the heart, which then
pumps it to the rest of the
body. Carbon dioxide-rich,
deoxygenated blood is
returned to the right side
of the heart and carried
back to the lungs for gas
exchange.

- **Nervous System:** The
  autonomic nervous
  system, in particular the
  respiratory centers in the
  brainstem, controls the
  respiratory system. These
  centers take information
  from different sensory
  receptors and modify the
  depth and pace of
  breathing accordingly. The
  control of breathing
  muscles including the
  diaphragm and intercostal
  muscles is another
  function of the neural
  system.

Breathing is made easier by the
interaction of the
musculoskeletal system with the

respiratory system. The chest cavity is expanded and contracted during inhalation and exhalation by the diaphragm, a dome-shaped muscle at the base of the lungs, and the intercostal muscles between the ribs. To make it easier for air to enter and exit the lungs, these muscles collaborate with the ribcage's skeletal structure.

- **Immune system:** In the fight against airborne diseases and foreign particles, the respiratory system serves as the first line of defense. In order to filter and trap dangerous chemicals, the respiratory system is lined with specialized cells and structures, including as cilia and mucus-producing cells. The immune system, which includes immune cells specific to the respiratory system, works to recognize and get rid of germs, lowering the risk of respiratory infections.
- **Endocrine System:** Hormones produced by the endocrine system have an

impact on respiratory function. For instance, the hormone adrenaline, which the adrenal glands release in reaction to stress or physical activity, can influence breathing rate and airway dilatation. Additionally, as shown in diseases like obesity or some endocrine disorders, hormonal imbalances can have an impact on respiratory function.

The digestive system's main jobs are to break down food and assimilate nutrients, but it also has structural similarities to the respiratory system. Both food and air can move via the pharynx, a shared route. When swallowing, food and liquid are kept out of the respiratory tract by the epiglottis, a tissue flap in the throat.

Skin, hair, and nails are all parts of the integumentary system, which works with the respiratory system to regulate body temperature. By exchanging heat and moisture with the environment during exhale, the respiratory system aids in the regulation of body temperature. The nasal passages and nose also assist in humidifying and filtering breathed air.

list of typical respiratory conditions

- **Asthma:** Asthma is a chronic disease marked by inflammation and airway constriction. It results in recurrent attacks of shortness of breath, chest tightness, coughing, and wheezing. Allergens, physical activity, respiratory illnesses, and environmental variables can all be asthma triggers.

- **COPD, also known as chronic obstructive pulmonary disease:** Chronic bronchitis and emphysema are two lung diseases that are part of the chronic obstructive pulmonary disease (COPD) group. It is generally brought on by repeated exposure to irritants like cigarette smoke or toxins from the workplace. Airflow obstruction brought on by

COPD results in symptoms including coughing up a lot of mucus, wheezing, and shortness of breath.

- **Pneumonia:** A lung infection typically brought on by bacteria, viruses, or fungus is known as pneumonia. It causes swelling and a buildup of fluid in the air sacs, which results in symptoms including coughing, fever, chest pain, and breathing difficulties. From moderate to severe, pneumonia can occur and frequently needs medical attention.

Inflammation of the bronchial tubes, which transport air to and from the lungs, is known as bronchitis. Both acute and chronic conditions are possible. The symptoms of acute bronchitis include coughing, chest congestion, and mucus production. Viral infections are typically at blame. A persistent cough that lasts for at least three months over the course of two consecutive years characterizes chronic bronchitis, which is frequently linked to smoking.

- **Flu**: A highly contagious viral respiratory ailment, influenza. It may result in symptoms including fever, weariness, body pains, coughing, sore throats, and nasal congestion. The flu can cause complications, including pneumonia, in severe cases.

- **Pulmonary Fibrosis:** The thickening and scarring of lung tissue is a hallmark of this progressive lung condition. This scarring makes it difficult for the lungs to expand and contract, which causes weariness, a dry cough, and shortness of breath. Pulmonary fibrosis can have an idiopathic (unknown) etiology could be brought on by things like being exposed to pollutants in the environment, using specific medications, or having underlying medical issues.

Sleep apnea is a sleep disorder marked by pauses in breathing while you're asleep. It happens when the neck muscles fail to keep the airway open, causing momentary pauses in breathing. Loud snoring, daytime tiredness, morning headaches, and difficulties focusing are some symptoms that may be present. Allergy to airborne allergens like pollen, dust mites, or pet dander causes allergic rhinitis, also referred to as hay fever. Sneezing, runny or stuffy nose, itching, and nasal congestion are some of the symptoms it causes.

Lung Cancer: The unchecked expansion of abnormal cells in the lungs is known as lung cancer. It may result in symptoms like unintentional weight loss, a chronic cough, chest pain, shortness of breath, and coughing up blood. Although non-smokers can also get lung cancer, smoking is the main risk factor.

I'll go into more depth about the first five because they are among the most prevalent ailments and can have a big influence on people's health and quality of life.

(1) Asthma

Lung damage from asthma is a frequent respiratory illness. Simply put, asthma is a disorder where a person's airways narrow and swell, making it challenging for them to breathe normally. The airways of someone who has asthma are more vulnerable to specific triggers. These triggers may include things like allergens (like pollen, dust mites, or pet dander), respiratory diseases, exercise, stress, or exposure to specific irritants (such smoke or potent scents), and they can differ from person to person. A person with asthma who is exposed to their triggers may experience tightening of the muscles surrounding their airways, swelling of the lining of their airways, and an increase in mucus production. The airways become more constricted as a result of the interaction of these factors, making it more difficult for air to enter and exit the lungs. A person with asthma may consequently have symptoms like wheezing (a whistling sound made during breathing), coughing (particularly at night or in the early morning), shortness of breath, and heaviness in the chest.

what causes asthma

Although the precise etiology of asthma is still unknown, it is thought to be a result of both hereditary and environmental factors. Here are some asthma-related probable causes and risk factors:

Asthma tends to run in families, which raises the possibility of a genetic susceptibility. Asthma risk may be increased by particular genetic variants. A family history of asthma does not, however, ensure that a person will ultimately get the ailment.

- **Environmental allergens:** Allergens are compounds that, in certain people, might cause an allergic reaction. Pollen, dust mites, pet dander, mold spores, and specific foods are some of the common allergens linked to asthma. These allergens can cause airway inflammation and asthma symptoms in people who already have the condition.

- **Respiratory Infections:** Respiratory infections, particularly viral illnesses like the common cold, can cause asthma symptoms to flare up or aggravate pre-existing asthma. A number of respiratory infections can irritate the airways, making them more sensitive and vulnerable to the symptoms of asthma.

- **Exposure to Irritants:** Some irritants and pollutants can aggravate asthma symptoms or raise the likelihood that someone will acquire asthma. Cigarette smoke, air pollution, chemical fumes, potent scents, and interior or outdoor contaminants are a few examples.

- **Factors related to the workplace:** Some work situations expose people to toxins that can exacerbate asthma symptoms or

perhaps cause it.
Chemicals, dust, gases,
and fumes are a few
examples of these
substances.

- **Obesity:** Asthma risk
  factors have been linked to
  obesity. Although the
  precise mechanisms
  causing the association
  between fat and asthma are
  not fully known, it is
  thought that the persistent
  low-grade inflammation
  linked to obesity may be a
  factor in the onset or
  exacerbation of asthma
  symptoms.
- **Other Factors:** Other
  factors that may cause
  asthma include early-life
  respiratory infections,
  secondhand smoke
  exposure, exposure to
  certain medications (like
  beta-blockers or NSAIDs),
  and hormonal changes in
  women (like those that
  occur during menopause
  or pregnancy).

It's vital to remember that
everyone has different asthma
triggers. What causes asthma

symptoms in one person might not in another. In addition, asthma may manifest up suddenly and without a known reason.

Asthma symptoms.

Asthma symptoms might differ from person to person in terms of severity and frequency. They may change over time even within the same person. Here are a few typical asthma symptoms:

- **Wheezing:** When air passes through constricted airways, it makes a whistling or high-pitched sound known as wheezing. It is a defining asthma symptom and is typically audible during exhale. However, occasionally wheeze can also happen while inhaling.
- **Dyspnea:** Dyspnea, another name for shortness of breath, is a sensation of being out of breath or having trouble breathing. Depending on how severe the asthma attack is, it can range from moderate to severe and happen while

moving around or even while at rest.

- **Coughing:** Persistent coughing is a typical asthma symptom. It might be more obvious at night or early in the morning. Asthma-related coughing often produces little phlegm or mucus and is dry and non-productive.
- **Chest Tightness:** Asthmatics frequently experience a feeling of pressure or tightness in the chest. This symptom may give the chest area the sensation of being squeezed or constricted.
- **Sleeping Problems:** Asthma symptoms can deteriorate at night, disrupting sleep. Sleep disruption brought on by coughing, wheezing, and shortness of breath can result in weariness and afternoon drowsiness.
- **Rapid Breathing:** Asthma symptoms, particularly those that are severe or that occur during an asthma attack, can

occasionally produce rapid and shallow breathing.

- **Increased Mucus Production:** Asthma can cause the airways to produce more mucus, which might feel congested or like phlegm in the throat or chest.

Keep in mind that not every asthmatic suffers each of these signs and symptoms. While some people may only occasionally have symptoms, others may deal with more severe or enduring symptoms. Furthermore, throughout time, both the intensity and frequency of symptoms can change, with times of symptom-free intervals and flare-ups brought on by numerous triggers.

Important methods for managing asthma: medical diagnosis:

- **Controller medication:** medicine used to prevent and manage asthma symptoms is known as a controller medicine. They include of long-acting beta-agonists, leukotriene modifiers, inhaled

corticosteroids, and
additional choices that
your doctor has
recommended.

- **Emergency medications**:
  When asthma symptoms
  or flare-ups occur, short-
  acting bronchodilators,
  commonly referred to as
  quick-relief or rescue
  drugs, are used to provide
  immediate relief. These
  drugs function by
  releasing the tension in the
  airway muscles and
  widening the airways.
- **Allergy medications:** If
  allergens are a factor in
  your asthma symptoms,
  your doctor may advise
  using nasal corticosteroids
  or antihistamines to help
  manage allergic reactions.

Action Plan for Asthma:
Create a unique asthma action
plan in collaboration with your
healthcare practitioner. This plan
will detail daily management
tactics, medication
administration, and what to do in
the event of asthma attacks or
symptoms that worsen.

You will be better able to spot triggers, react to them, change medication dosages as necessary, and know when to seek medical attention.

How to Recognize and Avoid Triggers:

Discover your unique triggers and take action to minimize their occurrence. Allergens (pollen, dust mites, pet dander), irritants (smoke, strong odors, chemicals), respiratory illnesses, and exercise are examples of common triggers.

Maintaining good indoor air quality requires maintaining clean interior settings, using dust mite covers on bedding, avoiding exposure to pet allergens, utilizing air filters, and making sure that sufficient ventilation is in place.

Regular Inspection:

Utilize a peak flow meter to routinely track your symptoms and peak flow values (a measurement of lung function). This might assist you in monitoring changes in the management of your asthma and modifying your therapy as necessary.

Maintain contact with your doctor for routine checkups to evaluate your asthma control, go over your treatment plan, and make any required modifications.

Choices for a Healthy Lifestyle:

Continually lead a healthy lifestyle that includes frequent exercise, a nutritious food, and enough sleep. Talk to your doctor about the best fitness program and any safety measures you should take to avoid developing exercise-induced asthma.

Avoid smoking and being around others who are smoking, as both can exacerbate the symptoms of asthma and raise the risk of complications.

Education and Assistance:

Learn about asthma, its causes, and how to take your medications. Attend asthma education sessions or sign up for support groups to hear from and learn from people who have the disease.

As accurate inhaler technique is necessary for efficient drug delivery, learn how to utilize inhalers and other asthma devices.

Because each person has a different type of asthma, it's essential to collaborate closely with your healthcare practitioner to create a personalized asthma management plan. To effectively manage asthma and lessen its influence on your everyday life, regular communication with your doctor and adherence to the recommended therapy are essential.

COPD, also known as chronic obstructive pulmonary disease, The lung condition known as chronic obstructive pulmonary disease (COPD) makes it challenging for a person to breathe. Since it is a chronic disorder, it usually gets worse with time.

COPD is essentially a mix of the two most common lung conditions, emphysema and chronic bronchitis. Let's examine each one in turn:

Chronic bronchitis is a disorder in which the lungs' airways (bronchial tubes) swell up and secrete an excessive amount of mucus. For at least three months throughout the course of two successive years, this results in a chronic cough and increased mucus production. Breathing becomes more difficult due to the inflammation and abundant mucus constricting the airways.

Emphysema: Emphysema is a disease in which the lungs' air sacs, or alveoli, suffer injury and lose their elasticity. During breathing, these air sacs are in charge of exchanging carbon dioxide and oxygen. Emphysema causes breathing difficulties and diminished lung function because the injured air sacs are less effective at transporting oxygen into the bloodstream.

Chronic obstructive pulmonary disease (COPD) causes

Long-term exposure to irritants that harm the lungs is the main cause of Chronic Obstructive Pulmonary Disease (COPD). The majority of instances of COPD are caused by smoking cigarettes, which is the main risk factor. However, COPD development might also be influenced by other causes. The following list of typical causes and risk factors:

- **Smoking:** Tobacco use, including both active smoking and secondhand smoke exposure, is the main contributor of COPD. Over time, the damaging compounds included in cigarette smoke irritate and inflame the lungs, harming the airways and air sacs.
- **Environmental Factors:** COPD risk can be increased by prolonged exposure to several environmental irritants and toxins. Long-term exposure to air pollution, chemical fumes, dust, and industrial contaminants are a few examples. COPD can also develop as a result of occupational exposure to materials including asbestos, silica, and coal dust.
- **Genetic Factors:** Genetic factors may occasionally contribute to the development of COPD. Early-onset COPD can result from a hereditary disease called alpha-1

antitrypsin deficiency. A protein that shields the lungs from harm has low levels or behaves abnormally in people with this impairment.

- **Infections of the respiratory tract:** Repeated or serious respiratory infections, particularly in children, can cause lung damage and raise the chance of developing COPD in later life. Chronic inflammation and scarring of the airways can be brought on by specific respiratory illnesses, such as repeated attacks of pneumonia.

Asthma: Although COPD and asthma are separate illnesses, long-term, uncontrolled asthma can raise the chance of developing COPD. Poorly controlled asthma can cause persistent inflammation, airway damage, and the onset of COPD-like symptoms as well as airflow restriction.

Not everyone who is exposed to these risk factors will get COPD, it is crucial to remember this.

There are different levels of individual susceptibility to lung injury and the onset of COPD. Additionally, elements including smoking frequency and duration, genetic susceptibility, and the presence of other medical disorders might have an impact on how severe COPD is.

Chronic obstructive pulmonary disease (COPD) symptoms

Chronic obstructive pulmonary disease (COPD) symptoms can range in severity and may appear gradually. The most typical signs are as follows:

One of the main signs of COPD is shortness of breath, sometimes known as dyspnea. It may begin as a moderate case of shortness of breath while engaging in physical activity, but as it gets worse, it may eventually happen even when at rest or doing very little. Some people may feel as though they are suffocating or are having trouble breathing.

- **Chronic Cough:** A chronic cough is one of the typical signs of COPD. Mucus or phlegm may come out of the cough, especially in the morning.

The cough could get worse and more regular over time.

- **Increased Mucus Production:** People with COPD frequently produce more mucus in their airways. As a result, you can experience chest congestion and frequently clear your throat or cough to get rid of the mucus.
- **Wheezing:** When you wheeze, you make a high-pitched whistling sound. It is brought on by the airways narrowing, which restricts the free movement of air.
- **Chest Tightness:** Some people with COPD may feel as though their chests are squeezed or under pressure. This could make it uncomfortable and make breathing more challenging.
- **Fatigue:** The greater effort needed to breathe as a result of COPD might make you feel tired or lack energy. Exhaustion may result from impaired

oxygen exchange caused by decreased lung function.

- **Weight Loss:** COPD patients who have severe stages may experience weight loss and muscular wasting. Unintentional weight loss may result from the increased energy demand for breathing paired with decreased hunger and less physical activity.

Methods for controlling Chronic Obstructive Pulmonary Disease (COPD)

Chronic Obstructive Pulmonary Disease (COPD) management calls for an all-encompassing strategy that incorporates medical care, lifestyle changes, and self-care techniques. The following are crucial elements in managing COPD:

Medications:

- **Bronchodilators:** By assisting in the relaxation of the airway muscles, these drugs improve airflow. Depending on how long they take to work, they can be either short-acting or long-acting.

In moderate to severe cases, bronchodilators are frequently used with inhaled corticosteroids to assist reduce inflammation in the airways.

Other Drugs: Other drugs, such as antibiotics (for respiratory infections) or mucolytics (to thin mucus), may be recommended depending on the patient's requirements and particular symptoms.

The rehabilitation of the lungs

Programs for pulmonary rehabilitation combine fitness instruction, knowledge, breathing exercises, and nutritional advice that are specifically designed for people with COPD. These initiatives aid in symptom management, physical functioning improvement, and quality of life improvement.

Therapy using Oxygen

Supplemental oxygen therapy may be administered when there are low blood oxygen levels. To increase oxygenation and reduce shortness of breath, it involves using oxygen through a mask or nasal cannula.

changes to one's way of life
The most crucial action in controlling COPD is to **stop smoking**. This may lessen symptoms and help the disease grow more slowly.
Lung Irritants Should Be Minimized: Limit exposure to substances such as secondhand smoke, air pollution, chemicals, and other lung irritants. When working with dangerous materials, use caution.
Immunizations: Annual pneumococcal and flu vaccinations are advised to avoid respiratory infections, which can exacerbate the symptoms of COPD.
Exercises for the lungs and breathing techniques:
Breathing techniques like pursed-lip breathing and diaphragmatic breathing can enhance breathing effectiveness and lessen shortness of breath.
Individualized physical activity can assist build stronger respiratory muscles and increase overall endurance. To choose the best exercises, speak with medical professionals.
A healthy way of life

Keep up a balanced diet full of fresh produce, whole grains, lean proteins, and other healthy foods. Nutritionally sound eating habits enhance general health and energy levels.

Drink plenty of water to keep your airways wet and thin your mucus.

To lower the risk of respiratory infections, practice proper hygiene.

Regular Follow-Up and Monitoring:

For the best management of COPD, regular check-ups with medical specialists are necessary to track the condition's development, change medications as necessary, and maintain compliance.

You can regularly check your lung function at home by using a peak flow meter or spirometer. It's essential to collaborate closely with medical providers to create a customized COPD management strategy and attend to particular demands. The symptoms of COPD can be managed effectively, exacerbations can be reduced, and overall quality of life can be raised.

3 Pneumonia

A typical and possibly dangerous lung infection is pneumonia. It happens when the air sacs in one or both lungs swell up and become irritated, producing fluid or pus that makes breathing difficult. Pneumonia is an infection that affects the lungs and can make you feel quite ill, to put it simply.

pneumonia causes

Numerous infectious organisms, including as bacteria, viruses, fungi, and parasites, are capable of causing pneumonia. The following are some typical pneumonia causes:

Infections caused by bacteria: Pneumonia is frequently brought on by bacteria. Streptococcus pneumoniae (pneumococcus), Haemophilus influenzae, Legionella pneumophila, Staphylococcus aureus, and Mycoplasma pneumoniae are the most typical bacterial pathogens that can cause pneumonia.

Another typical cause of pneumonia is viral infections, particularly in kids and during viral outbreaks. Adenoviruses, respiratory syncytial viruses (RSV), adenoviruses, and coronaviruses (particularly SARS-CoV-2, the virus that causes COVID-19) are common viral infections that can cause pneumonia.

Pneumonia can also be brought on by fungi, especially in people with compromised immune systems or those exposed to certain environmental factors. People who work in vocations that expose them to contaminated soil or bird droppings or who live in certain geographic areas tend to have fungal pneumonia more frequently. Examples of fungi that can cause pneumonia include Aspergillus species, Cryptococcus neoformans, and Histoplasma capsulatum.

When foreign things, such as food, drinks, vomit, or saliva, are aspirated into the lungs, aspiration pneumonia results. Dysphagia or a compromised gag reflex are two conditions that might lead to this. Numerous germs that are often found in the mouth or throat might cause aspiration pneumonia.

Pneumonia that is hospital-acquired or healthcare-associated: If a patient is receiving mechanical ventilation or has a compromised immune system, pneumonia may manifest during or after a hospital stay. Hospital-acquired pneumonia is typically brought on by more virulent bacteria, such as Pseudomonas aeruginosa or methicillin-resistant Staphylococcus aureus (MRSA). Pneumonia that is obtained outside of a hospital setting is referred to as "community-acquired pneumonia." Numerous infectious organisms, including as bacteria, viruses, and fungi, are capable of causing it.

It's crucial to remember that the causes of pneumonia might change based on things like age, general health, and location. For proper treatment recommendations and good infection management, identifying the precise cause of pneumonia is crucial.

The signs of pneumonia

Pneumonia symptoms can change based on the underlying cause, the severity of the infection, and the patient's general condition. The following list of pneumonia symptoms is typical:

Cough: One of the main signs of pneumonia is a persistent cough. The sputum's color can range from clear or white to yellow, green, or even crimson, and the cough may generate phlegm or pus.

temperature: Pneumonia frequently results in a high temperature, usually greater than 100.4°F (38°C). Chills, sweating, and a general feeling of being poorly may accompany the fever. Breathing might become challenging due to pneumonia's impact on the lungs, which impairs their capacity to exchange oxygen. Breathlessness is possible, especially while exerting yourself physically. Even breathing at rest might be difficult in severe cases.

Chest Pain: Chest pain can range in intensity from a minor discomfort to a strong, stabbing ache in people with pneumonia. When you move, cough, or take heavy breaths, the pain could get worse.

Weakness and exhaustion: The body's immunological reaction to pneumonia as well as the extra effort needed to breathe can result in weakness and exhaustion. You can experience energy loss and exhaustion.

Rapid Heartbeat and Rapid Breathing: The body tries to make up for the impaired lung function by quickening both the heartbeat and breathing. Your heart could seem to be racing more quickly than normal, and you might notice that your breathing quickens.

A bluish coloring of the lips, fingertips, or nails (cyanosis) may happen in severe cases or when oxygen levels in the blood are abnormally low. The cause of this is insufficient oxygenation. It's crucial to remember that different symptoms can range in severity and combination. Some people may experience more severe symptoms or problems, particularly those who have compromised immune systems or underlying medical issues. In senior people, symptoms like disorientation or changes in mental status may be more mild or unusual.

You must consult a doctor right away if you think you have pneumonia or exhibit symptoms including a persistent cough, a high temperature, trouble breathing, or chest pain. Effective management and the avoidance of pneumonia-related consequences depend on early identification and treatment.

Key methods for treating pneumonia

A combination of medical therapy, rest, and self-care techniques are used to manage pneumonia. Here are some effective treatments for pneumonia:

Medical diagnosis:

- **Antibiotics:** If bacteria are the cause of your pneumonia, your doctor may recommend taking antibiotics to help treat the illness. Even if you begin to feel better, it's crucial to take the recommended antibiotics exactly as instructed and finish the entire course of therapy.

- **Antiviral Drugs:**
  Antiviral drugs may be
  administered if the
  pneumonia was brought on
  by a viral illness, such as
  the flu. These drugs
  diminish the severity and
  duration of the symptoms
  while also lowering the
  viral load.

Hospitalization may be required
in extreme circumstances or if
you have underlying medical
issues. This enables close
observation, the delivery of
intravenous antibiotics or
antivirals, and, if necessary,
oxygen therapy.

Rest and Restoration

- **Get Lots of Sleep:** While
  your body battles the
  illness, it's crucial to rest
  and save energy. Avoid
  overworking yourself, and
  do things that will help
  you unwind and recover.

Stay Hydrated: To stay
hydrated, consume plenty of
liquids, such as water, herbal tea,
and clear soups. Dehydration is
avoided and mucus is thinned as
a result.

To prevent the infection from spreading to others, practice respiratory hygiene by covering your mouth and nose with a tissue or your elbow when you cough or sneeze.

support services

- **Pain relief:** Acetaminophen or nonsteroidal anti-inflammatory medicines (NSAIDs), which are available over-the-counter, can help reduce fever, chest pain, and discomfort brought on by pneumonia. Follow the dose instructions and, if necessary, seek medical advice.

- **Use a Humidifier:** You can reduce coughing and relax your respiratory passages by using a humidifier to provide moisture to the air or by having a steamy shower.

- **Avoid Smoking and Secondhand Smoke:** Smoking and secondhand smoke exposure can exacerbate symptoms and slow the healing process.

During and during the recuperation phase, it's crucial to avoid smoking and limit your exposure to smoke.

- **Follow Medication Instructions:** Use prescription drugs as instructed and pay attention to your doctor's instructions if you're given bronchodilators or mucolytics to help manage your symptoms.

Sustained Care:

- **Attend Follow-Up Appointments:** It's crucial to show up to any follow-up appointments that your doctor has set. They can evaluate your development, keep track of your healing, and modify your treatment plan as needed.

Keeping up with immunizations, such as the annual flu shot and the pneumococcal vaccine, can help prevent pneumonia and its complications.

4. Bronchitis

The respiratory ailment known as bronchitis is characterized by inflammation and irritation of the bronchial tubes, the lungs' airways. Simply put, bronchitis is an inflammation of the airways that enter and exit your lungs. Acute bronchitis and chronic bronchitis are the two main kinds of bronchitis.

Acute bronchitis is a short-term ailment typically brought on by a viral infection, such as the flu or the common cold. A persistent cough that produces phlegm or mucus, which might be clear, white, yellowish, or greenish in hue, characterizes it. Chest discomfort, a sore throat, a moderate temperature, weariness, and a general feeling of being poorly are possible additional symptoms. With rest and the right care, acute bronchitis often lasts for a few weeks before going away on its own.

Chronic Bronchitis: A more severe and protracted form, chronic bronchitis. A chronic cough that lasts for at least three months over the course of two consecutive years is what distinguishes it. Smoking and prolonged exposure to irritants like dust, pollen, or chemical fumes are frequently linked to chronic bronchitis. Excessive mucus production and a persistent cough are caused by the continuing inflammation and irritation in the bronchial tubes. Other signs and symptoms could include chest pain, exhaustion, recurring respiratory infections, wheezing, and shortness of breath. A more serious disorder known as chronic obstructive pulmonary disease (COPD) includes chronic bronchitis as one of its symptoms.

Excessive mucus is produced by the inflamed bronchial tubes in both types of bronchitis, which can obstruct the airways and make breathing more challenging. To open the airways and clear the mucus, this may cause coughing.

Why does bronchitis occur?

Depending on the type of bronchitis, many factors can contribute to it. The typical causes are listed below:

Chronic Bronchitis:

Acute bronchitis is most frequently brought on by viral infections, such as the same viruses that cause the flu or the common cold. These viruses can cause inflammation by infecting the bronchial passages.

Bacterial Infections: While less often than viral infections, acute bronchitis can occasionally be brought on by bacterial infections. After contracting a viral respiratory infection, bacterial bronchitis can develop as a secondary infection.

recurring bronchitis

Smoking tobacco, including cigarettes, cigars, and pipe smoking, is the main contributor of chronic bronchitis. Smoke irritates the bronchial tubes, which causes persistent inflammation and the formation of mucus.

Environmental Irritants: Chronic bronchitis can also be brought on by prolonged exposure to other irritants such air pollution, chemical fumes, dust, and specific industrial pollutants.

Genetic Factors: Some people may be more likely to develop chronic bronchitis as a result of genetic factors that influence how well their lungs and respiratory systems operate.

It's crucial to remember that bronchitis brought on by bacterial or viral illnesses can be communicable in both acute and chronic forms. When an infected individual coughs or sneezes, the viruses or bacteria that caused the infection might spread through respiratory droplets. However, smoking- or environment-related chronic bronchitis is not communicable.

Principal treatments for bronchitis

By changing your lifestyle and taking care to lower your risk of respiratory infections and irritants, you can prevent bronchitis. Here are some steps you can do to prevent this:

1. **Avoid Smoking and Secondhand Smoke:** If you smoke, quitting is the most important thing you can do to prevent bronchitis, especially chronic bronchitis. Smoking weakens the respiratory system and harms the lungs,

increasing your risk of developing respiratory illnesses. Reduce your exposure to secondhand smoke as well because it can irritate your bronchial tubes.

2. **Follow Good Respiratory Hygiene Procedures:** To lower the risk of respiratory infections, practice good respiratory hygiene procedures. These consist of:

-Regularly wash your hands with soap and water, paying particular attention before touching your face, chewing, or preparing meals.

-When soap and water are not available, use hand sanitizers.

-To stop respiratory droplets from spreading, cover your mouth and nose with a tissue or your elbow while coughing or sneezing.

-Properly dispose of used tissues. Reduce your exposure to environmental irritants that can irritate your lungs and bronchial tubes.

3. Avoid Environmental Irritants. Air pollution, dust,

chemical fumes, and other airborne particles may be among these irritants. Use the proper protective gear and adhere to safety procedures if you work in a workplace with high levels of irritants.

4 Strengthen Your Immune System: A healthy immune system can aid in the prevention of infections. Keep up a healthy way of life by:

-Eating a well-balanced diet full of fresh produce, healthy grains, lean meats, and other nutrients.

-Exercising frequently to improve general health and fortify your immune system.

-Getting enough sleep so that your body can recover and heal itself.

-Controlling stress levels because ongoing stress can impair immunity.

5 Maintain Recommended Immunizations: Maintain recommended vaccines, particularly for viral illnesses like influenza (flu) and pneumonia. Vaccinations can lower the risk of problems and help prevent several respiratory infections.

6 Maintain Good General Hygiene: To reduce the risk of illnesses, maintain good general hygiene. This comprises:
-Regularly disinfecting and cleaning surfaces that are regularly touched, such as doorknobs, light switches, and electronic gadgets.
-Staying far away from people who have respiratory infections. Your chance of getting bronchitis and other respiratory infections can be considerably decreased by implementing these preventive strategies into your lifestyle. It's always advisable to speak with a healthcare professional for individualized advice and guidance if you have any particular questions or medical conditions.

4. Flu or influenza

The respiratory illness influenza, more frequently referred to as the flu, is brought on by influenza viruses. It has an impact on the nose, throat, and even the lungs. The symptoms of the flu are typically more severe than those of the common cold.

The signs of influenza

Flu symptoms can vary from person to person, but typically include the following:

High fever: The flu frequently manifests as a high fever. It can range from mild to severe and is frequently one of the first symptoms.

Body pains and muscular pain: The flu frequently causes body aches and muscle pain, which can be severe and make moving about painful.

Extreme weariness and weakness can be brought on by the flu, which frequently leaves people feeling run down and unmotivated.

Headache: Headaches, which can range in severity from mild to severe, are frequent during the flu.

A sore throat is a typical symptom that frequently comes with discomfort or pain when swallowing.

Runny or stuffy nose: Nasal congestion brought on by the virus might result in a runny or stuffy nose.

Cough: A dry, lingering cough is another typical flu symptom. It could get worse over time and be accompanied by chest pain.

Sweating and chills: People who have the flu frequently feel sweating and chills, which are frequently accompanied by changes in body temperature. Although these symptoms are more frequent in children than adults, the flu can occasionally also cause other symptoms like nausea, vomiting, and diarrhea.

Important flu management strategies

You can take the important actions listed below to manage influenza (flu) and lessen symptoms:

- Drink plenty of water and get plenty of rest to help your body heal. Getting enough sleep improves your immune system's capacity to combat the illness. To stay hydrated and avoid dehydration, consume plenty of liquids, such as water, herbal tea, and clear broths.
- Over-the-Counter Drugs: Over-the-counter painkillers can help lower fever, ease body pains, and

relieve headaches. Examples include acetaminophen (Tylenol) and ibuprofen (Advil, Motrin). If you have any questions or underlying medical conditions, get medical advice and adhere to the dosage recommendations.

- Use over-the-counter medications to treat certain symptoms. For instance, saline nasal sprays or decongestants can relieve nasal congestion, while cough suppressants or expectorants can aid with coughing.

The best way to prevent the flu from spreading to others is to stay home from work, school, or other public areas until your fever has subsided for at least 24 hours without the aid of fever-reducers. When coughing or sneezing, cover your mouth and nose with a tissue or your elbow, and throw away used tissues right away.

Seek Medical Care: The majority of flu illnesses may be treated at home. However, some people may be more vulnerable to issues and need to visit a doctor. This covers young children, elderly people, pregnant women, those with long-term medical disorders (such heart disease, diabetes, or asthma), and people with compromised immune systems. Seek immediate medical attention if your symptoms increase or if you experience severe symptoms, such as breathing difficulties, persistent chest discomfort, confusion, or extreme dehydration.

Antiviral Drugs: If you are at a high risk of problems or are experiencing severe symptoms, your doctor may occasionally recommend antiviral drugs such oseltamivir (Tamiflu). If used during the first 48 hours following the onset of symptoms, these drugs can help lessen the intensity and length of the flu. If you seek medical attention, heed the advice and treatment schedule suggested by your healthcare provider. Based on your unique situation and medical background, they may offer extra advice.

Always remember that preventing the flu is the best course of action. The best approach to avoid getting the flu or to lessen how bad it is if you do is to receive a yearly flu shot. The flu can also be stopped from spreading by following good hygiene habits including routine hand washing, covering your mouth and nose while coughing or sneezing, and avoiding close contact with ill people.

Different Life Stages and Respiratory Health

Early life and childhood

- The respiratory system is still growing during infancy. The chance of respiratory problems can be increased by premature birth or exposure to specific risk factors.
- Lung development requires a critical period throughout childhood. Respiratory infections, asthma attacks, and allergies can all be made more likely by factors including exposure to secondhand smoke, allergens, and pollution

- By guaranteeing a smoke-free atmosphere, providing a clean and dust-free living space, and encouraging frequent physical exercise, you can help children's respiratory health.

Teenage years and early adulthood:

The respiratory system continues to develop during these phases. Risky habits like smoking, vaping, or exposure to contaminants in the environment, however, can have long-term repercussions on lung health.

- Inform teenagers and young adults of the risks associated with smoking and vaping. Encourage adopting a healthy lifestyle, which includes frequent exercise, a balanced diet, and avoiding environmental toxins.

Adulthood:

Maintaining good respiratory health in adulthood is essential for overall wellbeing. Asthma, chronic bronchitis, and occupational lung disorders are a few of the common respiratory conditions that might develop.

- Avoid smoking and being around people who are smoking. When working in dangerous areas, wear the proper respiratory equipment to save your lungs.
- Exercise regularly, keep up a healthy diet, manage stress, and have frequent check-ups to keep an eye on your lungs.

Older people:
The respiratory system naturally ages and changes. Breathing becomes harder as lung flexibility declines. Respiratory infections and chronic illnesses like COPD and pneumonia are more common in older persons.

- Maintaining a healthy lifestyle, using proper hygiene, receiving the required immunizations (such the flu and pneumonia shots), and avoiding exposure to respiratory irritants are all ways to promote respiratory health.

- Regular exercise, including breathing techniques and chest physical therapy, can support lung health and avert respiratory problems.

Pregnancy:

-Due to hormonal changes and increased oxygen demands, pregnancy might have an impact on respiratory health. Asthma and other pre-existing respiratory problems may need specific attention during pregnancy.

-To support respiratory health, pregnant women should receive regular prenatal care, adhere to their doctor's instructions, and maintain good general health.

The book "Small Steps, Great Gain: Adding Years to Your Lifespan" has examined the critical subject of respiratory health and how it affects our general wellbeing. We have explored the complexities of the respiratory system, the widespread respiratory conditions that impact millions of people worldwide, and the significance of taking a proactive approach to managing and

maintaining healthy lungs
throughout this book.
We now know that our quality of
life and respiratory health are
closely related, and that the
decisions we make every day can
have a big impact on how long
we live and how well our lungs
operate. Understanding the
respiratory system's architecture
and physiology has helped us
better grasp how our lungs
function and how crucial it is to
take care of them.
We have learned about the
devastating effects that common
respiratory illnesses including
bronchitis, pneumonia, chronic
obstructive pulmonary disease
(COPD), and asthma may have
on sufferers and their loved ones.
We have also seen the
effectiveness of information and
preventative steps in treating
these conditions and raising
people's quality of life.
The importance of lifestyle
variables in promoting healthy
lungs has been highlighted in the
book. We can significantly
improve and maintain the health
of our respiratory system by
adopting small but significant

behavioral changes like quitting smoking, avoiding environmental toxins, exercising frequently, using deep breathing techniques, and eating a balanced diet. We have also discussed the significance of early detection, getting the appropriate medical attention, and adhering to treatment schedules for respiratory disorders. We can take charge of our lung health and make wise decisions now that we are aware of the signs, causes, and treatment options for a variety of respiratory problems. The book "Small Steps, Great Gain: Adding Years to Your Lifespan" serves as a reminder that we have control over our respiratory health and that we can add years to our lives by making tiny but substantial efforts. Every breath we take is a priceless gift, and by taking care of and protecting our lungs, we can improve our general health and live longer, healthier lives that are also more enjoyable. May you be motivated and empowered by this book to put your respiratory health first, to make wise decisions, and to appreciate the simple actions that add up to big results. Let's set out on this adventure together, giving our lungs new life, and welcoming the limitless opportunities that are ours for the taking when we take control of our respiratory health.

Keep in mind that we have the chance to take care of our lungs, broaden our horizons, and leave a legacy of wellness with each and every breath. Small actions taken today can have a big impact tomorrow, extending our lives and allowing us to fully appreciate everything that life has to offer.

CHAPTER 5

Emotional and mental health.

The state of one's psychological and emotional health is referred to as their mental and emotional well-being. It includes a person's general mental health, including their thoughts, feelings, and actions, as well as their capacity to handle and adjust to the difficulties of life.

Cognitive activities including perception, thought, reasoning, and problem-solving are all included in mental well-being. It shows how mentally healthy we are, including how strong our emotions are, how confident we feel in ourselves, and how well we can handle stress. Our capacity to identify, comprehend, and regulate our emotions is a key component of emotional well-being. It entails being aware of our emotions, expressing them appropriately, and controlling our emotional reactions in diverse circumstances.

The Importance of Emotional and Mental Health

The Importance of Emotional and Mental Health

Our general health, happiness, and quality of life are strongly influenced by our mental and emotional well-being. They are crucial for the following reasons, which are all very important:

- **Enhanced Resilience:** People with resilience— the capacity to recover from failures, adapt to change, and flourish in the face of adversity—have a strong foundation of mental and emotional well-being. It gives us the emotional fortitude and coping skills need to deal with life's difficulties.

- **Better Relationships:** Our ability to interact with people is positively influenced by our mental and emotional health. We may create stronger, more meaningful connections, communicate clearly, and empathize with others' emotions when we are intellectually and emotionally balanced.
- Optimal performance in a variety of spheres of life, including job, school, and personal hobbies, depends on mental and emotional health. We can think creatively, make better decisions, and be more productive when our brains are clear, focused, and not overly stressed.
- **Overall Health and Well-Being:** Our

emotional and mental health are strongly correlated. Chronic stress, worry, and unresolved emotional difficulties have been linked to a number of health conditions, including immune system deterioration, digestive disorders, and cardiovascular diseases, according to research. Our entire health and longevity can be positively impacted by placing a high priority on our mental and emotional well-being.

- **Life Satisfaction:** Having a strong feeling of mental and emotional wellbeing helps one feel more fulfilled and satisfied with life. We are more likely to feel happy, enjoy life's events, and develop a feeling of meaning and purpose when we feel cognitively and emotionally in balance.

The Mind-Body Connection:

1. View from a holistic perspective: The term "mind-body connection"

describes the complex and reciprocal interaction between our mental and emotional well-being and our physical health. It acknowledges that both our mental and physical health can be affected by our ideas, feelings, beliefs, and attitudes.

2. Communication paths: The neurological system, endocrine system, and immune system are just a few of the paths through which the mind and body can exchange information. The release of stress hormones like cortisol, for instance, can have an effect on both mental and physical health.

3. **Influence of Thoughts and Emotions:** The body's physiological reactions are influenced by thoughts and emotions. Positive feelings and thoughts like thankfulness and joy can improve general wellbeing, whereas negative feelings and thoughts like stress and

anxiety can worsen physical health problems.

Health Effects of the Mind-Body Connection
Physical Fitness

1. The mind-body link is essential to understanding how the body reacts to stress. Long-term or persistent stress can cause imbalances in the body, raising the risk of illnesses like heart disease, digestive problems, and impaired immune system.

2. Immune System Functioning: Immune system responses are influenced by the mind-body relationship. Negative emotions and long-term stress can stifle immunological responses, rendering people more prone to sickness, whereas positive emotions and mental states have been linked to enhanced immune function.

3. The mind-body link has an impact on how we experience and perceive pain. Techniques like

relaxation, meditation, and
cognitive-behavioral
treatments can help control
pain by changing the
mind's perception of pain
signals. Emotional and
psychological elements
can regulate how we
perceive pain.

Mood and Mental Health

- **Emotional Control:** The
  mind-body connection
  shows that having a
  positive mental and
  emotional state has a big
  impact on overall health.
  Positive emotions and
  efficient stress
  management skills
  improve psychological
  well-being whereas
  negative emotions and
  ongoing stress can
  contribute to mental health
  issues including anxiety
  and depression.
- Psychosomatic symptoms:
  When emotional or
  psychological anguish
  appears as physical
  symptoms without a clear
  medical reason, this is an
  example of the mind-body

link in action. By using holistic strategies that take into account both mental and physical health, addressing these symptoms is made easier with an understanding of the mind-body relationship.

Personal Choices

- Health and Behavior: Lifestyle decisions that affect general health are influenced by the mind-body link. Diet, exercise, sleep, and substance use are all activities that can be influenced by mental and emotional health. Healthy decisions are influenced by positive mental and emotional states, whereas unhealthy behaviors may result from poor mental or emotional states.

- Self-Care and Wellness Practices: People can prioritize self-care activities that promote both mental and physical wellness by understanding the mind-body link. A healthy mind-body connection is fostered through practicing mindfulness, physical activity, relaxation techniques, and getting enough sleep.

Frequently held beliefs and stigmas around mental health

Commonly held beliefs and unfavorable attitudes that contribute to misperceptions, prejudice, and social prejudices concerning mental health disorders are what we mean when we discuss common myths and stigmas around mental health. These myths and stigmas can make it difficult for people with mental health issues to get the support they need, receive the correct care, and lead satisfying lives.

Misconceptions are unfounded assumptions or attitudes regarding mental health that are not backed by facts or reliable information. These misunderstandings may be the result of societal prejudices, cultural influences, a lack of education, or a general lack of knowledge about mental health conditions.

On the other side, stigmas are unfavorable opinions and notions about people who have mental health disorders. Stigmas frequently result in prejudice, social isolation, and the marginalization of those who are dealing with mental health issues. Stigmas can be pervasive and have an impact on a variety of facets of life, such as interpersonal relationships, employment prospects, access to healthcare, and general well-being.

Examples of widespread myths and stigmas relating to mental health include:

- Believing that having a mental illness is a sign of weakness or a defect in one's character.
- Believing that those who struggle with mental illness are dangerous or violent.
- Considering mental health issues to be merely a passing phase or attention-seeking activity.

- Linking mental health problems to a lack of motivation or willpower.
- Discriminating against those with mental health issues by labeling them as "crazy" or "unstable."
- Believing that people who struggle with mental illness are unable to live happy and productive lives.
- Consider assistance for mental health problems to be a sign of failure or weakness.

People who are dealing with mental health disorders may suffer as a result of these myths and stigmas, which frequently deters them from getting the help and care they require. A more inclusive and welcoming atmosphere that supports mental health and well-being for all people requires challenging these myths and eradicating stigmas.

Aspects Affecting Mental and Emotional Health

Understanding the numerous aspects that affect mental and emotional health can help people and communities promote mental

health in a proactive manner. It is feasible to develop a supportive environment that encourages resilience, effective coping mechanisms, and all-around wellbeing for everyone by addressing biological, environmental, psychological, and trauma-related aspects. **The following are some variables that affect mental and emotional health.**
Biological Constraints

- Genetics: Genetic factors may predispose someone to developing particular mental health issues. The likelihood of acquiring similar illnesses may be increased by a family history of mental disorders.
- Brain Chemistry and Structure: Neurotransmitter imbalances and structural abnormalities in the brain can be causes of mental health problems. For instance, depression has been associated with decreased serotonin levels.

- Physical Health: A person's physical health, which includes aspects like diet, exercise, and sleep, can have an affect on their mental and emotional health. A sound body helps a sound mind.

Environmental Elements

a. Childhood Experiences: Early life events like trauma, abuse, or neglect can have a big impact on a person's mental and emotional health later in life. A higher incidence of mental health disorders has been linked to adverse childhood experiences (ACEs).

b. Social Support: Good relationships, a solid network of friends and family, and a feeling of community can all help people feel more mentally and emotionally healthy. Social networks, family ties, and encouraging friendships are essential for psychological well-being in general.

c. Socioeconomic Factors: A person's mental and emotional health can be impacted by economic stability, access to education, career possibilities, and living situations. Disparities in socioeconomic status might affect mental health outcomes and increase stress.

d. Social and cultural factors: Cultural norms, values, and beliefs affect how mental health is viewed, comprehended, and dealt with. Well-being can be greatly impacted by stigma, discrimination, and social attitudes regarding mental health.

Psychiatric variables

a. Effective coping strategies, resilience, and problem-solving abilities all contribute to mental and emotional well-being. Strong coping mechanisms enable people to handle difficulties more skillfully.

b. Positive self-esteem and a sound feeling of one's own value are essential for both mental and emotional wellness. Positive self-perception and self-acceptance can benefit one's psychological well-being in general.

c. Cognitive Patterns: Mental and emotional health can be impacted by thought patterns and cognitive processes like biased thinking, negative self-talk, and distorted thinking. Individuals who use cognitive-behavioral strategies can confront and change unproductive thought patterns.

Life's Occasions and Trauma

a. Important Life Transitions: Major life changes like loss, divorce, career changes, or relocation can have an effect on a person's mental and emotional health. The ability to adjust to change and handle the stress brought on by life's events is crucial for preserving wellbeing.

b. Traumatic Experiences: Trauma can have long-lasting repercussions on a person's mental and emotional health, whether it be physical, emotional, or psychological. Support and care that is trauma-informed are essential for rehabilitation and healing.

c. Chronic Stress: Long-term exposure to chronic stress, such as that brought on by work-related stress or the demands of caring, can have an adverse effect on one's mental and emotional health. Creating efficient stress management techniques is essential for preserving overall wellness.

Techniques for Overcoming Emotional and Mental Challenges

Awareness and Acceptance of Oneself

- Understanding Mental and Emotional issues: Having an awareness of one's mental and emotional issues is the first step in conquering them. Gaining self-awareness makes it easier to spot trends, triggers, and the particular problems that require attention.

- Acceptance: It's important to accept one's mental and emotional challenges without condemnation or blame of oneself. Acceptance paves the way for a kind and forgiving attitude toward oneself.

Getting Expert Assistance and Support

- Therapy and counseling: Attending therapy or counseling can give you useful tools and ways to handle and get through emotional and mental difficulties. A safe environment for emotion exploration, coping mechanism development, and perspective expansion is provided through professional assistance.

- Medication: To treat some mental health issues in specific situations, a doctor's prescription for medication may be required. Determining the best drug alternatives can be aided by speaking with a psychiatrist or other medical expert.

- Support Groups and Peer Networks: Connecting with people who have gone through comparable struggles or joining support groups can provide a sense of community, comprehension, and shared coping mechanisms. Peer support groups can offer important emotional support and useful guidance.

Creating Coping Mechanisms

- strategies for Dealing with Stress: Learning and using

strategies for dealing with stress, such as deep breathing exercises, mindfulness exercises, meditation, and relaxation techniques, can help control emotions and lessen stress.

- Healthy Lifestyle Options: Making healthy lifestyle choices can have a favorable effect on one's mental and emotional health. This entails engaging in regular exercise, eating a balanced diet, getting enough sleep, and minimizing or avoiding substances that may be harmful to one's mental health.

- **Building Resilience:** Developing resilience enables people to overcome obstacles and recover from setbacks. Building resilience entails practicing optimistic thinking, problem-solving techniques, adaptability, and requesting help when required.

Building Supportive Environments and Positive Relationships

- Relationships that Nurture: Positive, encouraging relationships are crucial for one's mental and emotional health. A robust support network is created by fostering meaningful and healthy relationships with family, friends, and the larger community.
- Setting Boundaries: It's important to set boundaries in your interactions with others and to prioritize your own needs. To preserve emotional well-being, it entails understanding personal boundaries and successfully communicating requirements.
- Making a Supportive Environment: Making a supportive environment involves limiting exposure to toxic influences, setting up a secure and tranquil physical area, and

partaking in enjoyable and fulfilling activities.

Self-care and mindfulness exercises

- Setting Self-Care as a Priority: Self-care activities customized to one's needs aid in rest and renewal. This can include things like taking up a hobby, going outside, cultivating self-compassion, and doing things that are enjoyable and relaxing.
- Meditation and mindfulness: Including meditation and mindfulness exercises in everyday routines improves self-awareness, lowers stress levels, and cultivates a sense of serenity. Techniques for mindfulness assist people in being present, observing their thoughts and feelings without passing judgment, and developing resilience.
- Seeking Joy and Meaning: Finding joy, meaning, and a feeling of purpose in one's activities can help

one's mental and emotional health. It encourages a sense of fulfillment and enjoyment to pursue interests, passions, and hobbies that are consistent with one's values and worldview.

It takes time, persistence, and a thorough strategy that considers all facets of wellbeing to overcome mental and emotional difficulties. Individuals can negotiate their obstacles, develop resilience, and enjoy increased mental and emotional well-being by combining self-awareness, professional assistance, coping mechanisms, caring connections, and self-care routines.

Long-Term Maintenance of Mental and Emotional Well-Being

Long-term mental and emotional well-being takes self-care, introspection, and a dedication to your total wellness. It is a journey that never ends. You may encourage resilience, promote better mental health, and enjoy a higher sense of fulfillment and happiness by adopting the ideas I'm about to share into your daily life.

Creating Healthful Habits

- Self-Care practice: Establish a regular self-care practice that consists of exercises that encourage unwinding, reducing stress, and having fun. This can involve indulging in enjoyable hobbies or pastimes, getting enough sleep, exercising regularly, and practicing mindfulness.

- Aim for balance in all aspects of your life, such as your work, relationships, and personal duties. Setting achievable goals, using time wisely, and upholding boundaries can all assist to avoid burnout and advance wellbeing.

- Set healthy boundaries in relationships and circumstances that could affect your mental and emotional wellbeing. Put yourself first and express your needs clearly to keep a healthy balance in your relationships and daily life.

Building Support Networks and Positive Relationships

- Maintaining Relationships: Surround yourself with wholesome and encouraging people. Spend time and energy cultivating and sustaining positive relationships with loved ones who support and promote your wellbeing.
- Seek Social assistance: In difficult times, reach out to your social networks for assistance. Don't be afraid to ask for help from others if you need emotional support, direction, or just someone to talk to. Getting involved in online forums or support groups can also give people a sense of belonging.
- Empathy & Kindness Training: In your relationships with others, practice kindness and empathy. Kindness-related activities enhance your wellbeing and sense of

fulfillment while also helping others.

Constant Learning and Personal Development

- Lifelong Learning: Take part in ongoing education and personal development. Engage in mental stimulation through reading, going to workshops, picking up new skills, or looking into educational opportunities. This encourages growth and a sense of success.
- Emotional intelligence can be developed by improving self-awareness, effective emotion management, and interpersonal and empathy abilities. Relationship management, conflict resolution, and improved self and other understanding are all made easier by having emotional intelligence.
- Goal-setting: Establish worthwhile objectives that are compatible with your values and desires. Having specific goals and

pursuing them gives one a sense of direction, motivation, and fulfillment.

Maintaining Mental Health as a Priority

- Checking in frequently will help you monitor your mental and emotional health. Check in with yourself, consider your emotions, and take proactive measures to resolve any indications of imbalance or distress.
- Include mindfulness and stress management practices in your everyday routine. To manage and reduce stress, practice stress-reduction methods including deep breathing, meditation, and relaxation exercises.
- Monitor Yourself-Talk: Be aware of your ideas about yourself and try to dispel any negative or low-self-esteem ones. Practice self-affirmations, self-encouragement, and self-compassion.

Making a Friendly Environment

- Make a safe and encouraging physical environment by designing it to encourage wellbeing. Make sure the areas where you live and work are tidy, well-organized, and encouraging of productivity.

- Digital Well-Being: Create wholesome digital habits by establishing time limits for screen usage, using technology with awareness, and avoiding distressing or upsetting content. Create a stress-reduction and mental health-supportive online environment.

- When necessary, get professional assistance if you are dealing with persistent or escalating mental health issues. To meet your unique requirements, mental health specialists can offer direction, support, and evidence-based interventions.

In the course of life, the state of
our mental and emotional health
is of utmost importance. It is
only by taking care of our inner
selves that we can fully realize
our potential for a happy and
satisfying life. This book's
chapter, "Small Steps, Great
Gain: Adding Years to Your
Lifespan," has focused on the
enormous influence of mental
and emotional health on our
entire quality of life. We have the
ability to improve our lives and
nurture permanent happiness by
focusing on this essential
component of who we are.
We started with comprehending
the meaning of mental and
emotional well-being and its
importance. We understood that
the two types of health—mental
and physical—are interdependent
and serve as the cornerstone of
our general well-being. We
dispelled widespread myths and
stigmas about mental health in an
effort to build a culture that is
more forgiving and welcoming.
We investigated how our ideas,
emotions, and physical health are
closely related as we dug deeper
into the mind-body relationship.

By understanding this relationship, we may make comprehensive decisions that promote both our mental and physical health. We came to understand the significant impact that genetics, environment, and individual experiences have on our mental health.

We also looked at methods for overcoming emotional and mental obstacles. We can overcome challenges, find healing, and progress through growing self-awareness, getting aid from an expert, and coming up with smart coping mechanisms. In this journey, we stressed the value of healthy relationships, self-care, and resilience so that we could empower ourselves to face challenges head-on and live happy, fulfilling lives.

Maintaining long-term mental and emotional health became an important priority. We may promote a long-lasting sense of well-being by developing healthy habits, cultivating great connections, and placing a high priority on our mental health. We realized that sustaining our

mental and emotional balance requires self-care, lifelong learning, and the development of supporting settings.
Let's accept these teachings and make a commitment to applying them to our daily activities.
Every decision we make, every choice to put our mental and emotional health first, has an impact that goes well beyond just ourselves. We contribute to a world that is healthier and more compassionate as we take care of our inner selves..

CHAPTER 6

CANCER PREVENTION
What is cancer?
Cancer is a disease that develops when the body's cells begin to proliferate and reproduce uncontrollably, to put it simply. Normal cell division and reproduction help us develop, repair injuries, and replace worn-out cells in our bodies. Cancer, however, is an example of where this mechanism fails.

Our bodies are made up of small building blocks called cells in every component. These cells have a lifespan and particular tasks. Old or damaged cells die off and are replaced by new cells in a healthy body. However, as cancer progresses, specific cells start to divide and expand too quickly, resulting in the formation of a tumor—a mass of aberrant cells.

The two types of tumors are benign and malignant. Non-malignant benign tumors often do not spread to other body areas and are not cancerous. Often, they can be removed or treated without much damage.

Malignant tumors, on the other hand, can infect adjacent tissues and spread to other areas of the body through a process known as metastasis. This is what makes cancer such a risky condition. Lungs, breasts, the colon, the skin, and many other body organs are just a few of the places where cancer can develop. varied cancers have varied signs, prognoses, and treatments. It's crucial to remember that not all lumps or tumors in the body are malignant; some may really be benign growths.

various cancers

There are numerous distinct forms of cancer, each of which develops in particular bodily cells or tissues. The following is a list of some prevalent cancer types:

- Breast cancer is a type of cancer that develops in the breast tissue and primarily affects women, however it can also affect men.
- Lung cancer is a type of lung cancer that commonly results from smoking but can also affect non-smokers.
- Colorectal cancer is a type of cancer that typically begins as polyps in the lining of the intestines and spreads to the colon or rectum.
- Male prostate cancer is a type of cancer that often spreads slowly and primarily affects elderly men.
- Skin cancer is a type of cancer that develops in skin cells and is frequently

brought on by ultraviolet (UV) radiation from the sun or tanning booths. Basal cell carcinoma, squamous cell carcinoma, and melanoma are the three primary forms.

- Bladder cancer is a type of cancer that develops in the bladder and is frequently linked to smoking and exposure to specific toxins.

- A blood or bone marrow cancer called leukemia is characterized by a fast generation of aberrant white blood cells. Acute lymphoblastic leukemia (ALL), acute myeloid leukemia (AML), chronic lymphocytic leukemia (CLL), and chronic myeloid leukemia (CML) are a few of the different kinds of leukemia.

- Lymphoma: A type of cancer that affects the immune system's lymphatic system. Hodgkin lymphoma and non-Hodgkin lymphoma

are the two main kinds of
lymphoma.
- Pancreatic cancer is a type
  of cancer that arises in the
  pancreas, a gland in the
  abdomen that creates
  hormones like insulin and
  digesting enzymes.
- Ovarian cancer is a type of
  cancer that develops in the
  ovaries, the female
  reproductive organs in
  charge of egg production.
- Cancer that starts in the
  cervix, the lower portion
  of the uterus, known as
  cervical cancer, is
  frequently brought on by
  specific HPV strains.

Cancer that develops in the
kidneys, which are the organs in
charge of filtering waste from the
blood.

**What are the risk factors and
causes?**

Depending on the type of cancer,
there may be different causes and
risk factors. Here are some
typical causes and risk factors
linked to the growth of cancer,
though:

- Age: As people get older,
  their risk of getting cancer

rises. Older persons are more likely to be diagnosed with several different types of cancer.

- Gene mutations that have been passed down through families can raise the chance of acquiring a particular type of cancer. It's crucial to remember, too, that only a small portion of malignancies are primarily brought on by inherited genetic abnormalities.

- Environmental conditions: Cancer risk can be raised by exposure to specific environmental substances and conditions. These may consist of:

Carcinogens: The risk of cancer can be raised by chemicals and compounds from tobacco smoke, air pollution, asbestos, pesticides, certain chemicals in the workplace, and other sources.

Radiation: Medical imaging tests that use radiation, occupational radiation exposure, or excessive ultraviolet (UV) radiation exposure from the sun or tanning beds can all raise your chance of developing cancer.

Habits and Lifestyle Decisions: Some lifestyle choices can lead to a higher risk of cancer. These consist of:

Use of tobacco products: Smoking or using tobacco products increases the chance of developing a number of cancers, including bladder, lung, mouth, and throat cancers.

Unhealthy Diet: Consuming a diet heavy in red and processed meats, saturated fats, processed foods, and little in the way of fruits, vegetables, and fiber may raise your chance of developing some cancers, including colon cancer.

Lack of Exercise: Sedentary lifestyles with little to no exercise have been linked to a higher risk of developing a number of cancers.

Regular and heavy alcohol use can raise the chance of getting some malignancies, including breast, liver, mouth, throat, and esophageal cancer.

Hormonal Factors: Certain cancers are more likely to develop when there are hormonal abnormalities or exposure to hormones. For instance, extended estrogen exposure without a progesterone balance can raise the risk of breast cancer. persistent Inflammation: Long-term exposure to irritants, certain autoimmune illnesses, or persistent infections can all contribute to chronic inflammation in the body, which raises the risk of some cancers. It's crucial to remember that a person's presence of one or more risk factors does not guarantee that they will get cancer. While some people with many risk factors may never acquire cancer, many people with no known risk factors nonetheless contract the disease. Understanding these risk factors, however, can assist people in making wise lifestyle decisions, adopting preventive measures, and going through the proper screening to find cancer early, when treatment is most successful.

Statistics and prevalence
Here are some statistics and prevalent information on cancer:

- Global Cancer Incidence:
  The World Health
  Organization (WHO)
  reports that cancer is one
  of the main causes of
  mortality worldwide, and
  that over the next 20 years,
  there will likely be an
  increase of around 50% in
  the number of new cases.
Common Types: Breast, lung,
colorectal, prostate, and stomach
cancers are the most frequently
diagnosed cancers worldwide.
- Deaths from cancer:
  Around the world, cancer
  is a major cause of death.
  With an estimated 9.9
  million deaths expected
  worldwide in 2020, cancer
  will overtake
  cardiovascular diseases as
  the second largest cause of
  mortality.
- Regional Variations:
  Cancer mortality and
  incidence rates might
  differ from region to
  region. Developed nations
  typically have greater
  cancer incidence rates
  because of things like
  aging populations and risk

factors related to lifestyle.
However, because of the
lack of resources for
healthcare, early
identification, and
treatment, cancer mortality
rates are typically greater
in developing nations.
Breast cancer is the most
prevalent type of cancer in
women worldwide. Breast cancer
incidence rates have been rising
recently, in part because of
improved diagnostic methods
and changing lifestyle factors.

- Lung cancer: For both men
  and women, lung cancer is
  the primary cause of
  cancer-related deaths
  worldwide. Although it is
  strongly linked to tobacco
  use, nonsmokers can also
  get lung cancer from other
  risk factors such contact
  with secondhand smoke,
  environmental toxins, or
  workplace dangers.

The third most prevalent cancer
diagnosed worldwide is
colorectal cancer, which also
encompasses colon and rectal
cancer. It affects both men and
women and is frequently linked

to lifestyle choices such poor eating habits, inactivity, and obesity.

Skin cancer is one of the most curable types of cancer, including melanoma and non-melanoma varieties. Skin cancer risk is increased by exposure to ultraviolet (UV) radiation from the sun or artificial sources like tanning beds.

Cancer survival rates might vary based on the kind and stage of the disease as well as the availability of prompt and efficient therapies. Numerous malignancies now have higher survival rates thanks to improvements in early diagnosis and treatment, but there are still problems, particularly with advanced or metastatic cancers.

methods for preventing cancer

Even while cancer can't always be prevented, making certain lifestyle decisions and taking preventative steps can greatly lower the risk of getting the disease. Here are some essential measures to help fight cancer:

- Don't Smoke or Use Tobacco Products: One of the most crucial stages in cancer prevention is to abstain from all tobacco use. Smoking has been linked to several cancers, including bladder, esophagus, oral, and throat cancers. At any age, stopping smoking is advantageous.

- **Adopt a Healthful Diet:** Consume an array of fruits, vegetables, whole grains, and lean proteins as part of a balanced diet. Reduce your intake of processed and red meats, saturated fats, and sweets. To take advantage of their antioxidant effects, eat a range of bright fruits and vegetables.

- **Maintain a Healthy Weight:** Cancers such as breast, colorectal, renal, and pancreatic are all more likely to develop in people who are overweight or obese. Utilize a healthy diet and consistent exercise to work toward reaching and maintaining a healthy weight.

- **Regular Physical Activity:** Aim for 75 minutes of intense exercise or 150 minutes of moderate-intensity aerobic activity each week. Regular exercise can reduce the risk of developing some malignancies, such as breast, colon, and lung cancer.

The chance of developing skin cancer rises with prolonged exposure to the sun's damaging UV radiation. By seeking out shade, donning protective clothing, applying sunscreen with an SPF of 30 or higher, and avoiding indoor tanning, you can protect your skin.

- Get vaccinated and engage in responsible sexual behavior since several STDs, such as hepatitis B and the human papillomavirus (HPV), can raise the chance of developing certain malignancies. Practice safe sex, get an HPV vaccine, and if you're at risk, think about getting a hepatitis B shot.

- **Limit Alcohol Consumption:** Drinking too much alcohol has been associated to a higher risk of developing a number of cancers, including oral, liver, breast, and colorectal cancer. Limit your alcohol consumption or don't drink at all.
- Minimize your exposure to environmental carcinogens such asbestos, benzene, formaldehyde, and other chemicals and pollutants to prevent getting cancer. If you operate in a field where occupational carcinogen exposure may occur, abide by safety regulations and take the appropriate safeguards.
- Regularly Screen and Check Yourself: Regular cancer screenings for breast, cervical, colorectal, and prostate cancer can aid in the early detection of the disease, when therapy is most effective. Observe the screening

recommendations according on your age, gender, and family history.

- **Maintain a Healthy Lifestyle:** Prioritize your general well-being, get enough sleep, and efficiently manage your stress. Keep a positive outlook, ask for help when you need it, and partake in activities that advance your mental and emotional wellbeing.

Keep in mind that while taking these precautions can dramatically lower your risk of getting cancer, they cannot guarantee that you won't. It's crucial to get advice from medical specialists, adhere to suggested practices, and have regular checkups in order to keep an eye on your health and spot any early indications of cancer. Let's keep in mind that every decision we make matters as we get to the end of this journey of baby steps towards a lifetime of cancer prevention. With each nutritious meal, each daily activity, and all the measures we take, we get closer to a time

when cancer won't be a problem.
We have the ability to control
our futures and design a life that
is as healthy and long-lasting as
possible by arming ourselves
with knowledge and taking
action.

Not only can incorporating these
simple measures into our daily
life help prevent cancer, but it
also shows our devotion to our
loved ones and to ourselves. It is
a statement that we respect our
health and are prepared to make
the necessary adjustments in
order to live a life that is full of
vitality and wellness.

May you use this book as a
beacon of light as you strive to
live a life free from cancer. May
these modest steps result in
significant improvements in your
quality of life and the number of
years you live, as well as in the
quantity and vitality of those
years. Let's take control of our
health one tiny step at a time by
accepting the power we each
possess.

Cheers to preventing cancer,
good health, and the amazing
years that lay ahead!